汉英对照

心电图教学图谱

（第二版）

Chinese-English

Electrocardiograms for Education

2nd Edition

刘 霞 编著

Liu Xia

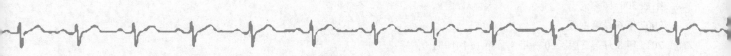

上海科学技术出版社

Shanghai Scientific & Technical Publishers

图书在版编目（CIP）数据

汉英对照心电图教学图谱 / 刘霞编著 . —2 版 . —上海：
上海科学技术出版社，2015.8（2023.4 重印）
ISBN 978−7−5478−2652−2

Ⅰ.①汉… Ⅱ.①刘… Ⅲ.①心电图 – 图谱 Ⅳ.
① R540.4−64

中国版本图书馆 CIP 数据核字（2015）第 108165 号

汉英对照心电图教学图谱（第二版）
Chinese-English Electrocardiograms for Education 2nd Edition

刘霞　编著

上海世纪出版（集团）有限公司
上 海 科 学 技 术 出 版 社　出版、发行
（上海市闵行区号景路 159 弄 A 座 9F−10F）
邮政编码 201101　www.sstp.cn
浙江新华印刷技术有限公司印刷
开本 889×1194　1/24　印张 9.5
字数 300 千字
2007 年 6 月第 1 版
2015 年 8 月第 2 版　2023 年 4 月第 16 次印刷
ISBN 978−7−5478−2652−2/R·913
定价：19.80 元

内 容 提 要

  本书为《汉英对照心电图教学图谱》的修订版。在上一版的基础上,本版依据国内临床诊断学的要求,采用汉英对照的形式,不仅详细描述了正常和异常心电图的最新诊断标准和形成机制,而且收录了典型心电图和一些疑难心电图的案例,并对其特征加以简明扼要的讲解,重点突出,图谱中需注意的异常部分通过标示着重指出,可使读者一目了然,易于掌握。本书可满足医学院校各学制的教学需求,也可为临床医生,尤其是内科医生所参考。

前　言

　　心电图问世至今已经有110多年的历史，是一门古老的学科。心电图曾经是心脏疾病诊断中仅有的两项检查方法之一，而今仍是临床上最为常见的检查方法，其检测范畴除心脏病学外，还涉及其他医学学科。每一位医学生在学习临床诊断学时都必须掌握心电图的基础知识。另外，心电图作为一项基本技能，也是各项考试中的重要组成部分。本书的特点之一是按照临床诊断学中心电图章节的内容和要求，系统地选用典型的心电图图例，并附上形象的图解，详细说明心电图上的特点和形成原理，旨在帮助医学生在学习理论知识的同时，提高对心电图图形的认识能力。本书的特点之二是中英文对照，便于医学生在学习心电图的同时，熟悉心电图的专业英文词汇，有利于今后医学英文文献的学习。本书的特点之三是在临床诊断学的基础上，拓展了国际公认的心电图新概念，有利于心电图新知识的普及。

　　本书图谱主要来自笔者的长期积累，部分由本科室同事提供，在此表示衷心感谢。本书的制图力求经典和精致，笔者为此付出了很多时间，在此对丈夫和儿子的理解和支持表示衷心感谢。

　　对心电的认识是无止境的，期盼各位读者对书中的心电图提出更多的宝贵意见，我的邮箱地址是 liuxia9110@163.com。

　　让我们一起认识变化无穷的心电图！

上海交通大学医学院附属瑞金医院心脏科

刘　霞

2015年5月

Preface

Since the invention of electrocardiogram (ECG), the study of it has marked a lengthy history of 110 years. ECG used to be one of the only two methods of diagnosing heart diseases, and it remains the most widely used even today, with its scope of examination ranging from cardiology to other medical fields. Every medical student, when studying the course of "Clinical Diagnostics," encounters some rudimentary knowledge of ECG. Meanwhile, ECG is also an important component of all kinds of standardized testing as a basic skill to be mastered by medical students. The ECG content in this book is highly correlated with the content of "Clinical Diagnostics." Selecting typical ECG examples and providing vivid diagram to illustrate the ECG characteristics and elucidate the formation mechanisms in a systematic way, this book is designed to help students develop ECG interpretation skills while gaining a theoretical background. It is written in both languages to familiarize students with the medical terms often used in the profession, benefiting future examination of references and literatures in English. Building upon the material of "Clinical Diagnostics," this book introduces new concepts recognized internationally in an effort to spread the most updated knowledge on ECG.

The ECG examples provided in this book mainly come from my own accumulation over the years. Some are provided by my colleagues, for whom I am very much thankful. Much time has been devoted to perfecting the illustration used in this book, and I would like to thank my husband and son for their continuing understanding and support.

The path toward understanding ECG is an infinite one. Thus, I look forward to comments and suggestions regarding the ECG used in this book. My email address is liuxia9110@163.com.

Let's begin our journey of understanding the ever-changing ECG!

Cardiology Department of Ruijin Hospital

Shanghai Jiaotong University Medical School

Liu Xia

May, 2015

目　录
Contents

第一章 心电图基本知识

Chapter 1　　**ABC of Clinical Electrocardiography**

心电图是从体表上记录心动周期中心脏的电活动。心电图仪采集和放大心肌组织除极和复极的微小电活动，并转化成波和段的图形。正常时，心脏的电活动起源于窦房结，由窦房结发出的冲动，首先激动右房，然后激动左房。窦房结的冲动在激动心房的同时，经房室结、希氏束和心室内传导系统（希－浦氏系统），最后激动左右心室。这一心脏节律称为正常窦性心律。

一、电极和导联

常规心电图需要10个电极，4个安放在肢体，6个安放在胸前。肢体电极组合构成6个肢体导联（Ⅰ、Ⅱ、Ⅲ、aVR、aVL和aVF导联），从垂直面观察心脏。6个胸前电极构成6个胸前导联（V1至V6导联），从水平面观察心脏。由此组成了常规12导联。

1. 双极肢体导联

- Ⅰ：RA(−)和LA(+)；
- Ⅱ：RA(−)和LL(+)；
- Ⅲ：LA(−)和LL(+)。

2. 加压单极肢体导联

- aVR：RA(+)和［LA + LL］(−)；
- aVL：LA(+)和［RA + LL］(−)；
- aVF：LL(+)和［RA + LA］(−)。

3. 胸前单极导联

Electrocardiography (ECG) is recording of the electrical activity of the heart on skin during each heart beat. ECG device detects and amplifies tiny electrical changes generated by depolarization and repolarization of the cardiac muscle, and translates them into a curve. In a normal heart, the cardiac impulse originates from the sinus node and spreads throughout the atria to activate the atria. After completion of the atrial activation, the impulse reaches and passes through the atrioventricular (A–V) node, and then travels through the His bundle, the right and left bundle branches, the left anterior and left posterior fascicles and the Purkinje fibers (His-Purkinje system) to activate the ventricles. This cardiac rhythm is termed normal sinus rhythm.

Electrodes and leads

For a routine ECG, 10 electrodes are attached, four to the limb and six to the chest wall. The information from the limb electrodes is combined to produce the six limb leads (Ⅰ, Ⅱ, Ⅲ, aVR, aVL, and aVF), which investigate the heart in the vertical plane. The six precordial leads (V1 to V6) investigate the heart in the horizontal plane. The information from these 12 leads is combined to form a standard ECG.

1. Bipolar limb leads (frontal plane)

- Ⅰ: RA(−) to LA(+);
- Ⅱ: RA(−) to LL(+);
- Ⅲ: LA(−) to LL(+).

2. Augmented unipolar limb leads (frontal plane)

- aVR: RA(+) to [LA and LL](−);
- aVL: LA(+) to [RA and LL](−);
- aVF: LL(+) to [RA and LA](−).

3. Unipolar (+) precordial leads (horizontal plane)

- V1: right sternal edge, 4th intercostal space;
- V2: left sternal edge, 4th intercostal space;
- V3: between V2 and V4;

- V1：胸骨右缘第四肋间；
- V2：胸骨左缘第四肋间；
- V3：V2和V4导联之间；
- V4：锁骨中线第五肋间；
- V5：腋前线V4导联水平；
- V6：腋中线V4导联水平。

（RA=右上肢；LA=左上肢；LL=左下肢）

二、心电图的组成和正常值

心电图是曲线形成的线图，由波和段组成。正负转折的称为波，两波之间的直线称为段。心电图上的组成成分被命名为P、Q、R、S、T和U，见图1。

1. P波代表右心房和左心房的顺序除极。正常值：

- Ⅰ和Ⅱ导联直立；
- aVR导联倒置；
- 时间<120 ms；
- 振幅<0.25 mV。

2. QRS波代表左右心室除极，通常左右心室同步被激动。正常值：

- Ⅱ导联和左胸导联主波向上；
- aVR和V1导联主波向下；
- 胸前导联由主波向下转为主波向上（见图2）；
- QRS波时间：60~100 ms，代表心室除

- V4: mid-clavicular line, 5th space;
- V5: anterior axillary line, horizontally in line with V4;
- V6: mid-axillary line, horizontally in line with V4.

(RA=right arm, LA=left arm, LL=left foot)

The components of the ECG and the normal values

A normal ECG is a curve with waves or complexes and segments. A wave is a single deflection turned either positive or negative, and a complex comprises of consecutive deflections. A segment is a distance between two waves or complexes. The letters that mark the various components of the ECG are P, Q, R, S, T and U (see Fig. 1).

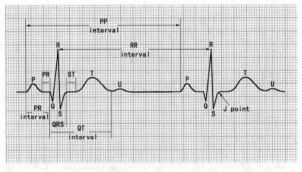

图1　心电图波和段的组成

Fig. 1　Components of the ECG

1. P wave: represents the sequential depolarization of the right and left atria. Normal values:

- upright in leads Ⅰ and Ⅱ;
- inverted in lead aVR;
- < 120 ms in duration;

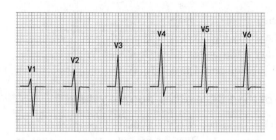

图2　胸前导联QRS波形态

Fig. 2　Patterns of QRS complex in precordial leads

极时间。

3. ST段位于J点和T波开始,代表心室除极结束和复极开始。正常值:位于基线或轻微移位,参考的基线为PR段或TP段。

4. T波代表心室复极。正常值:通常和同导联QRS波主波方向一致。

- Ⅰ、Ⅱ和V3~V6导联直立;
- aVR导联倒置,V1通常也倒置;
- Ⅲ导联可以倒置。

5. U波形成机制不清,许多心电图上不可见。

6. PR间期从P波开始至QRS波开始,代表心房开始除极至心室开始除极。在这间期中电活动在房室结、希氏束、束支、分支和浦氏纤维中传导。正常值:120~200 ms。

7. QT间期从QRS波开始至T波终末,代表心室除极和复极时间。推荐值:350~450 ms。

QT间期随心率变化而变化,心率缓慢,

- < 0.25 mV in amplitude.

2. QRS complex: represents the right and left ventricular depolarization, normally the ventricles are activated simultaneously. Normal values:

- upright in lead Ⅱ and in left precordial leads (V5 and V6);
- inverted in leads aVR and V1;
- QRS complex changes from mainly negative to mainly positive in precordial leads (see Fig. 2);
- QRS duration: width of QRS complex, 60 ~ 100 ms in duration, represents the duration of ventricular depolarization.

3. ST segment: between the J point and the beginning of the T wave, represents the period between the end of ventricular depolarization and the beginning of repolarization.

Normal values: lies in the baseline (isoelectric) or slightly above or below it, either the PR or TP segment is used as the reference baseline.

4. T wave: represents the ventricular repolarization.

Normal values: usually follows the QRS complex in orientation in the same lead.

- upright in leads Ⅰ and Ⅱ and in V3 ~ V6;
- always inverted in leads aVR and often in lead V1;
- can be inverted in lead Ⅲ .

5. U wave: origin for this wave is not clear. Many ECGs have no discernible U wave.

6. PR interval: from beginning of P wave to beginning of QRS complex, represents onset of the atrial depolarization to onset of the ventricular depolarization. During this time the electrical impulse is conducted through the A–V node, the bundle of His, the bundle branches, the fascicles and the Purkinje fibers.

Normal values: 120 ~ 200 ms in duration

7. QT interval: from beginning of QRS complex to end of T wave, represents the duration of ventricular depolarization and repolarization. General guide: 350 ~ 450 ms.

QT间期延长,因此测量时应参照心率变化。实际应用中常将QT间期通过Bazett's公式进行心率修正:QTc=QT/$\sqrt{RR}$(s)。

8. PP间期为心房周期,代表心房频率。正常值:60~100次/min。

9. RR间期为心室周期,代表心室频率,正常时心室频率等于心房频率。

三、心脏电轴

心脏电轴是反映心室除极和复极在垂直面上的综合方向。参考Ⅰ导联方向,向上偏移用负值,向下偏移用正值。正常心电轴的范围为:−30° ~ 90°之间(见图3)。−30°以外为电轴左偏,大于90°为电轴右偏。很多方法可以计算心脏电轴,简单的方法是目测Ⅰ、Ⅱ和Ⅲ导联的QRS波主波方向,若Ⅰ、Ⅱ和Ⅲ导联主波向上,一般电轴不偏,见表1。

表1 心脏电轴的估测

	正 常	右 偏	左 偏
Ⅰ导联	正向	负向	正向
Ⅱ导联	正向	正向或负向	负向
Ⅲ导联	正向或负向	正向	负向

更为精确的计算电轴至少需要2个肢体导联,常用的有Ⅰ和Ⅲ导联或aVF导联。测量R波和S波的振幅,求其代数和,然后将代

The duration varies with the heart's rate: the slower the rate the longer the QT interval. When measuring the QT interval the rate must be taken into account. Bazett's correction is used to calculate the QT interval corrected for heart rate (QTc): QTc=QT$\sqrt{RR}$ (s).

8. PP interval: duration of the atrial cycle, represents an indicator of atrial rate. Normal values: 60 ~ 100 bpm.

9. RR interval: duration of the ventricular cycle, represents an indicator of ventricular rate. The ventricular rate equals the atrial rate in normal.

Cardiac Electrical Axis

The cardiac electric axis refers to the mean direction of the ventricular depolarization wave in the vertical plane, measured with lead Ⅰ as a zero reference point. An axis lying above this line is assigned a negative number, and an axis lying below the line is assigned a positive number. The normal range for the cardiac axis is between −30° ~ 90° (see Fig. 3). An axis lying beyond −30° is termed left axis deviation, whereas an axis >90° is termed right axis deviation. Several methods can be used to calculate the electrical axis. The simplest method is by inspection of leads Ⅰ, Ⅱ, and Ⅲ as Tab. 1:

Tab. 1 The Estimation of Cardiac Electric Axis

	Normal	Right axis deviation	Left axis deviation
Lead Ⅰ	Positive	Negative	Positive
Lead Ⅱ	Positive	Positive or negative	Negative
Lead Ⅲ	Positive or negative	Positive	Negative

A more accurate way to calculate the axis uses at least two of the bipolar leads, normally leads Ⅰ and Ⅲ or aVF. Count from the baseline to the top and bottom of the R and S waves to determine the

数和画在导联轴上，作一垂线。两垂线相交点，与电偶中心0点相连，即为所求的心电轴，与Ⅰ导联电轴之间的偏移角度，即为心电轴的度数，详见图例2和3。

height (amplitude) of each wave. Subtract the two heights (algebraic sum). Then plot a point at hexaxial diagram according to this difference and draw a perpendicular line of the lead axis through the point. The two lines from the two leads intersect. Draw a line through this intersection point to the origin, the angel between the line and the lead Ⅰ axis represents the electrical axis deviation angel. This issue will be discussed in more detail in following articles (case 2 and 3).

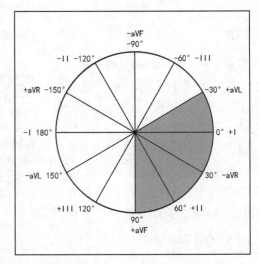

图3　心脏电轴（灰色部分为正常心脏电轴的范围）

Fig.3　Cardiac electric axis（grey is the normal range for the cardiac axis）

第二章　典型心电图案例及其解析

Chapter 2　**The Characteristics and Interpretation of Electrocardiograms**

图例1　正常心电图

Case 1　Normal Sinus Rhythm ECG

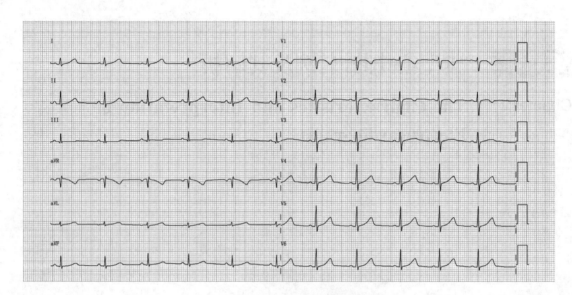

心电图特点

1. 心率：67次/min；PR间期：140 ms；QRS波时间：85 ms；QT/QTc间期：430/450 ms；QRS波电轴：70°。

2. P波在Ⅰ和Ⅱ导联直立，在aVR导联倒置。QRS波在Ⅰ、Ⅱ和左胸导联主波向上，在aVR和V1导联主波向下；胸前导联由主波向下转为主波向上。ST段位于基线或轻微移位。T波在Ⅰ、Ⅱ和V3～V6导联直立，在aVR导联倒置。

ECG Characteristics

1. HR: 67 bpm; PR: 140 ms; QRS D: 85 ms; QT/QTc: 430/450 ms; QRS axis: 70°.

2. P waves are upright in leads Ⅰ and Ⅱ, and inverted in lead aVR. QRS complexes are upright in leads Ⅰ, Ⅱ and in left precordial leads (V5 and V6), and inverted in leads aVR and V1; QRS complexes change from mainly negative to mainly positive in precordial leads.ST segments are at the baseline or slightly above or below it.T waves are upright in leads Ⅰ, Ⅱ and in V3 ~ V6, and inverted in lead aVR.

心电图诊断与解析

诊断：正常心电图。

解析：常用的心电图记录走纸速度是25 mm/s，测量PP间期或RR间期，可以用于计算心率。心率=60 秒/(PP间期或RR间期)。心电图上各导联P波和QRS波的识别见图1-1。QRS波需要再细分和命名，第一正向波命为R波，其前负向波命为Q波，其后负向波命为S波。在S波后若有第二个正向波，命为R′波。若为单一的负向波，命为QS波。大写字母代表波幅高（大于0.5 mV），小写字母代表波幅低（小于0.5 mV）。虽然如此命名，但无论有无Q波或S波，代表心室的波统称为"QRS"波。QRS波命名见图1-2。

ECG Interpretation

Normal sinus rhythm ECG.

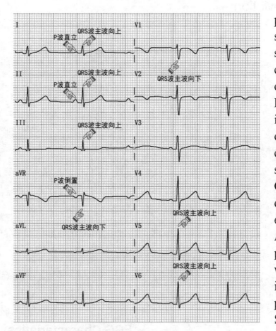

图1-1　心电图各波的识别

Fig. 1-1　Identification of the waves in ECG

Generally, the ECG paper is running at a standard speed of 25 mm/s. The heart rate can be calculated by measurement of the PP or RR interval: HR=60 s / (PP or RR interval). Identification of the P waves and QRS complexes in 12-lead ECG shows in Fig. 1-1. The QRS complex needs further dissection. The first upright deflection is an R wave. A negative deflection that precedes the R wave is a Q wave, and one that follows is an S wave. If a second positive wave follows the S wave, it will be called R′ (R prime) wave. When the ventricular complex has only a single negative deflection without any positive waves, it is described as a QS complex. Convention allows the use of capital letters (Q, R, S) for large amplitude waves (0.5 mV or more) and lowercase letters (q, r, s) for small amplitude waves (less than 0.5 mV). However, regardless of the waves it contains, any ventricular complex is referred to as thc "QRS complex." Fig. 1-2 shows how to mark the QRS complex.

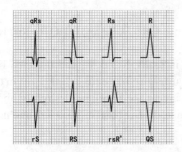

图1-2　QRS波的命名

Fig. 1-2　Nomenclature of the QRS complex

图例2　电轴左偏

Case 2　Left Axis Deviation

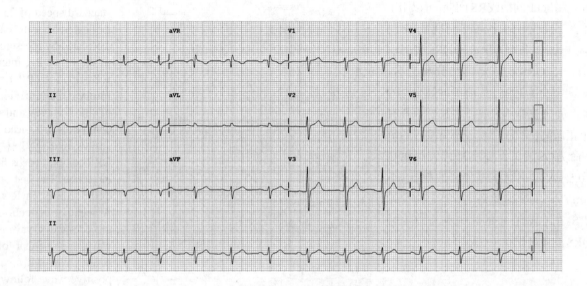

心电图特点

1. 心率：78次/min；PR间期：188 ms；QRS波时间：99 ms；QT/QTc间期：368/419 ms；QRS波电轴：−40°。

2. P波在Ⅰ和Ⅱ导联直立，在aVR导联倒置。QRS波在Ⅰ导联主波向上，在Ⅱ和Ⅲ导联主波向下。ST段位于基线或轻微移位。T波在Ⅰ、Ⅱ和V3～V6导联直立，在aVR导联倒置。

ECG Characteristics

1. HR: 78 bpm; PR: 188 ms; QRS D: 99 ms; QT/QTc: 368/419 ms; QRS axis: −40°.

2. P waves are upright in leads Ⅰ and Ⅱ, and inverted in lead aVR.QRS complexes are upright in lead Ⅰ, and inverted in leads Ⅱ and Ⅲ .ST segments are at the baseline or slightly above or below it. T waves are upright in leads Ⅰ, Ⅱ and in V3～V6, and inverted in lead aVR.

ECG Interpretation

Sinus rhythm, left axis deviation.

心电图诊断与解析

诊断：窦性心律；电轴左偏。

解析：心脏电轴测量方法见图2-1。在心电图Ⅰ和Ⅲ导联上，从基线测量R波和S波的振幅，求其代数和，Ⅰ导联=2.5 mm（0.25 mV），Ⅲ导联=-3.5 mm（-0.35 mV），见图2-1。然后，将代数和画在导联轴上，作一垂线。两垂线相交点与电偶中心0点相连即为所求的心电轴，与Ⅰ导联电轴之间的偏移角度（-40°）即为心电轴的度数（见图2-2）。偏移角度超过（小于）-30°则为电轴左偏，常见于左前分支阻滞和部分左心室肥大。

Fig. 2-1 shows the calculation of the electrical axis. Count from the baseline to the top of the R waves and the bottom of S waves to obtain the amplitudes in leads Ⅰ and Ⅲ. Take the difference of the amplitudes in both leads: lead Ⅰ =2.5 mm (0.25 mV) and lead Ⅲ = -3.5 mm (-0.35 mV), see Fig. 2-1. On the hexaxial diagram, plot the differences on their respective lead axis and draw a line perpendicular to the axis through each plotted point. The two lines from the two leads intersect. Draw a line from the origin (0 point) through this intersection point. The angel (-40°) between the line and Ⅰ axis represents the electrical axis deviation angel (see Fig. 2-2). An angle beyond (smaller than) -30° indicates left axis deviation, which commonly occurs in left anterior fascicular block and in certain cases of left ventricular hypertrophy.

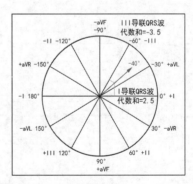

图2-2　心脏电轴测量

Fig. 2-2　Calculation of the cardiac electrical axis

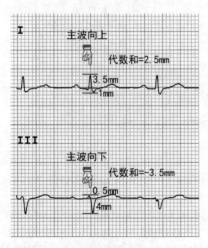

图2-1　R和S波的代数和

Fig. 2-1　Sum of the amplitudes of R waves and S waves

图例3　电轴右偏

Case 3　Right Axis Deviation

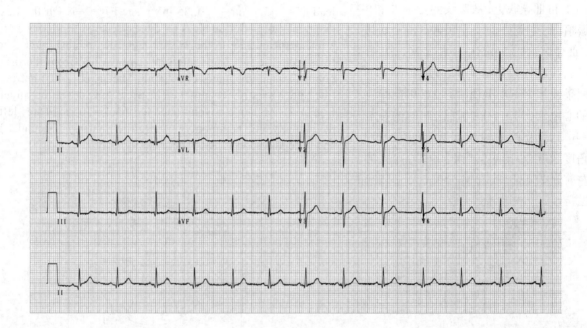

心电图特点

1. 心率：76次/min；PR间期：140 ms；QRS波时间：78 ms；QT/QTc间期：368/414 ms；QRS波电轴：99°。

2. P波在Ⅰ和Ⅱ导联直立，在aVR导联倒置。QRS波在Ⅰ导联主波向下，在Ⅱ和Ⅲ导联主波向上。ST段位于基线或轻微移位。

ECG Characteristics

1. HR: 76 bpm; PR: 140 ms; QRS D: 78 ms; QT/QTc: 368/414 ms; QRS axis: 99°.

2. P waves are upright in leads Ⅰ and Ⅱ, and inverted in lead aVR.QRS complexes are inverted in lead Ⅰ, and upright in leads Ⅱ and Ⅲ.ST segments are at the baseline or slightly above or below it.T waves are upright in leads Ⅰ, Ⅱ and in V3 ~ V6, and inverted in lead aVR.

T波在Ⅰ、Ⅱ和V3～V6导联直立，在aVR导联倒置。

心电图诊断与解析

诊断：窦性心律；电轴右偏。

解析：心脏电轴测量方法见图3-1。Ⅰ和Ⅲ导联R波和S波的代数和，Ⅰ导联＝−1 mm（−0.1 mV），Ⅲ导联=8 mm（0.8 mV），见图3-1。所求的心电轴与Ⅰ导联正侧段之间的偏移角度=99°（见图3-2）。电轴＞90°即为电轴右偏，常见于左后分支阻滞和右心室肥大。

ECG Interpretation

Sinus rhythm, right axis deviation

Fig. 3-1 illustrates again the calculation of electrical axis. The differences in amplitudes of R and S waves are equal to −1 mm (−0.1 mV) in leads Ⅰ and 8 mm (0.8 mV) in leads Ⅲ, see Fig. 3-1. The resulting angle is equal to 99° (see Fig. 3-2). An angle greater than 90° indicates right axis deviation, which commonly occurs in left posterior fascicular block and right ventricular hypertrophy.

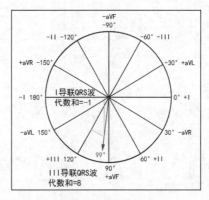

图3-2　心脏电轴测量

Fig. 3-2　Calculation of the cardiac electrical axis

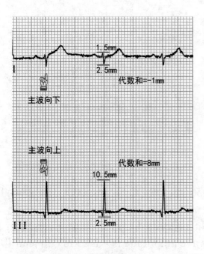

图3-1　R和S波的代数和

Fig. 3-1　Sum of the amplitudes of R waves and S waves

图例 4　右心房肥大 (异常)

Case 4　Right Atrial Enlargement (Abnormality)

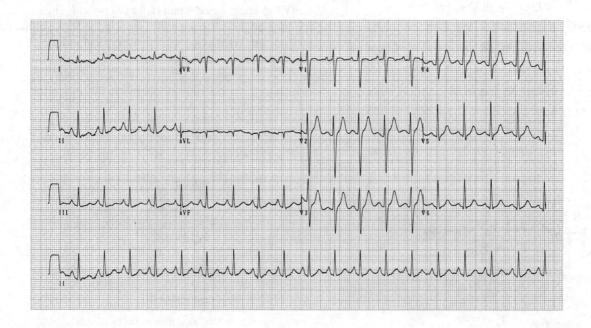

心电图特点

1. 心率：113次/min；PR间期：150 ms；QRS波时间：92 ms；QT/QTc间期：328/449 ms；QRS波电轴：74°。

2. P波在 I 和 II 导联直立，aVR导联倒置；心率 > 100次/min。II 导联P波振幅 > 0.25 mV。

ECG Characteristics

1. HR: 113 bpm; PR: 150 ms; QRS D: 92 ms; QT/QTc: 328/449 ms; QRS axis: 74°.

2. P waves are upright in leads I and II , and inverted in lead aVR; HR is > 100 bpm. P wave amplitude is > 0.25 mV in lead II .

ECG Interpretation

Sinus tachycardia,right atrial enlargement (abnormality).

The right atrial depolarizes before the left atrial, thus right

心电图诊断与解析

诊断: 窦性心动过速; 右心房肥大(异常)。

解析: 右心房除极先于左心房, 因此右心房肥大时仅产生P波前半部分改变, P波总时间不延长。右心房的解剖位置和除极方向是向下和向前, 因此右心房电势增加在下壁导联(Ⅱ, Ⅲ和aVF导联)和前壁导联产生高尖的P波。右心房肥大的诊断标准是Ⅱ导联P波振幅>0.25 mV和(或)V1导联P波振幅>0.15 mV。Ⅱ导联上高尖P波识别见图4-1。根据AHA/ACC/HRS "心电图标准化与解析建议" ("AHA/ACC/HRS建议"): "在心电图学早期已经认识到左右心房的解剖学异常或生理学异常均可引起心电图P波的异常。P波异常通常由多重因素所致, 且很难分辨究竟是何种因素引起, 因此, 更为模糊的术语如'左心房异常'和'右心房异常'更适合用来描述心房的异常"[1]。国内尚未确定相关术语。

atrial enlargement only affects the first portion of the P wave without prolonging its overall duration. The anatomical location and the direction of excitation of the right atrium are such that its forces are oriented inferiorly and anteriorly. An increase in the right atrial potential is therefore usually associated with the tall P waves in the inferior (Ⅱ, Ⅲ and aVF) and anterior leads (V1 and V2). Diagnostic criteria for right atrial hypertrophy are the P wave amplitude > 0.25 mV in lead Ⅱ and/or > 0.15 mV in lead V1. Fig. 4–1 shows the tall P wave in lead Ⅱ. According to "AHA/ACCF/HRS Recommendations for the Standardization and Interpretation of the Electrocardiogram" ("AHA/ACCF/HRS Recommendations"), "Abnormalities in the P wave that are related to anatomic or physiological abnormalities in the right or left atrium have been recognized since the early years of electrocardiography. Because the effects of these several factors on the P wave may often appear in combination and may not be distinguishable, the less specific terms left atrial abnormality and right atrial abnormality are preferable." [1] The term is yet to be determined in China.

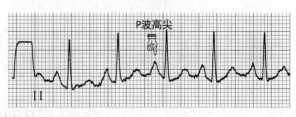

图4-1　P波高尖

Fig. 4–1　Tall P wave

图例 5　左心房肥大（异常）

Case 5　Left Atrial Enlargement (Abnormality)

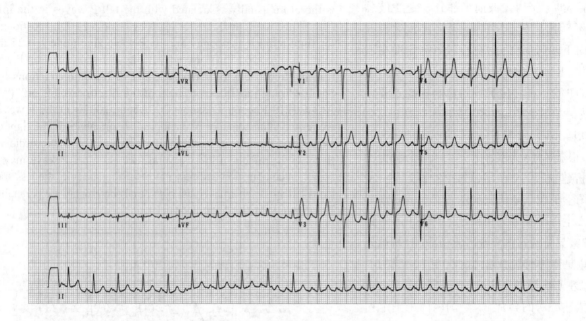

心电图特点

1. 心率：115 次/min；PR 间期：142 ms；QRS 波时间：70 ms；QT/QTc 间期：304/420 ms；QRS 波电轴：27°。

2. P 波在 I 和 II 导联直立，在 aVR 导联倒置；心率 >100 次/min。P 波时间 >120 ms，双峰，峰间距 >40 ms。V1 导联 Ptf 绝对值 >

ECG Characteristics

1. HR: 115 bpm; PR: 142 ms; QRS D: 70 ms; QT/QTc: 304/420 ms; QRS axis: 27°.

2. P waves are upright in leads I and II, and inverted in lead aVR; HR is > 100 bpm. P wave duration is > 120 ms, double-peaked with the inter-peak duration > 40 ms. P-terminal force in lead V1 is > 0.04 mm·s.

0.04 mm·s。

心电图诊断与解析

诊断：窦性心动过速；左心房肥大（异常）。

解析：左心房除极形成P波的中后部分，因此左心房肥大时产生P波中后部分改变。除极时间延长和左心房除极电势增加，可延长P波时间，并使P波呈双峰或有切迹。P波增宽＞120 ms，双峰，峰间距＞40 ms，提示左心房肥大。P波在V1导联中常呈双向，右心房在前，电势向前，形成P波起始正向波；左心房在后，电势向后，形成P波终末负向电势，称之为"终波终末电势（Ptf）"。V1导联Ptf值＝负向波振幅（mm）×时间（s），绝对值＞0.04 mm·s，也提示左心房肥大。Ⅱ导联P波双峰和V1导联Ptf增大见图5-1。根据"AHA/ACC/HRS建议"：更为模糊的"左心房异常"这一用词更适合用来描述[1]该情况。国内尚未确定相关术语。

ECG Interpretation

Sinus tachycardia, left atrial enlargement (abnormality).

The left atrial depolarization contributes to the middle and terminal portions of the P wave. Thus changes from left atrial hypertrophy are seen in the later portion of the P wave. The prolongation of depolarization and increase of the left atrium forces can both cause a prolonged P wave, double-peaked or notched in shape. The P wave duration is >120 ms, notched or double-peaked with inter-peak duration > 40 ms, suggests left atrial enlargement. The P wave in lead V1 is often biphasic. The early right atrial forces anteriorly give rise to an initial positive deflection, while the left atrial forces posteriorly produce a later negative deflection, termed as "P-terminal force (Ptf)". The value of "Ptf" is the amplitude (mm) × the duration (s) of the negative deflection in lead V1. The absolute value > 0.04 mm·s also suggests left atrial enlargement. Fig. 5-1 shows doubled-peaked P wave in lead Ⅱ and increased absolute value of "Ptf" in lead V1. According to "AHA/ACCF/HRS Recommendations", the less specific term left atrial abnormality is preferable.[1] The term is yet to be determined in China.

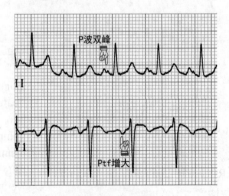

图5-1　P波双峰和Ptf增大

Fig. 5-1　Double-peaked P wave and increased absolute value of "Ptf"

图例6　左心室肥大

- -

Case 6　Left Ventricular Hypertrophy

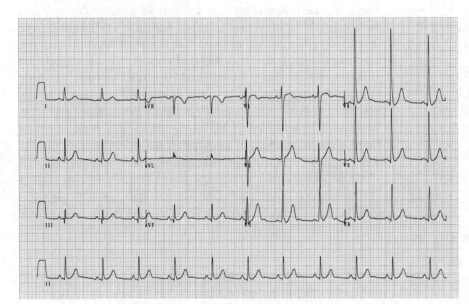

ECG Characteristics

1. HR: 66 bpm; PR: 142 ms; QRS D: 104 ms; QT/QTc: 404/423 ms; QRS axis: 53°.

2. R wave amplitude in lead V5 is > 2.5 mV, $R_{V5} + S_{V1} > 3.5$ mV.

3. QRS complex duration is > 100 ms.

ECG Interpretation

Sinus rhythm, left ventricular hypertrophy.

The left ventricle is anatomically at the left and backward location, and the excitation is directed towards the left. Many ECG criteria have been suggested for the diagnosis of left ventricular hypertrophy, but none is universally accepted. According to their corresponding ECG features, these criteria are classified as voltage or non-voltage. The most commonly used diagnostic criteria is based on the QRS voltages (amplitude) generated by the left ventricle. In a normal heart, the left ventricle myocardium is thicker than the right ventricle myocardium. The left ventricle is thus the major ventricle and the forces of left ventricular activation dominate the balance in a normal heart. Left ventricular hypertrophy exaggerates this natural dominance in the QRS voltages, which leads to increased R waves amplitude in leads facing the left ventricle wall (I , aVL, aVF, V5 and V6), and increased S waves

心电图特点

1. 心率：66次/min；PR间期：142 ms；QRS波时间：104 ms；QT/QTc间期：404/423 ms；QRS波电轴：53°。

2. V5导联R波振幅>25mV，$R_{V5}+S_{V1}>3.5$mV。

3. QRS波增宽 > 100 ms。

心电图诊断与解析

诊断：窦性心律；左心室肥大。

解析：解剖上，左心室位于心脏的左后方，除极方向向左。许多诊断标准用于诊断左心室肥大，但无一项是被公认的。根据左心室肥大的心电图特点，诊断标准可分为电压标准和非电压标准。测定左心室产生的QRS波电压值（振幅）是诊断左心室肥大最常用的标准。正常心脏的左心室心肌明显厚于右心室，左心室电势占优势。左心室肥厚或扩大后，可使左心室优势更为突出，引起面向左心室的导联（Ⅰ、aVL、aVF、V5和V6）中QRS波振幅增加，而背对左心室的导联（V1和V2）S波振幅加深（见图6-1）。肢体导联电压标准包括：Ⅰ导联R波振幅>1.5 mV，aVL导联R波振幅>1.1 mV，aVF导联R波振幅>2.0 mV，以及$R_Ⅰ+S_Ⅲ>2.5$ mV。胸前导联电压标准包括：V5或V6导联R波振幅>2.5 mV，$R_{V5或V6}+S_{V1}>3.5$ mV。近来，$R_{aVL}+S_{V3}>2.8$ mV（男性）或>2.0 mV（女性），称为"Cornell电压"的诊断标准已用于临床。QRS波电压的测量见图6-2。

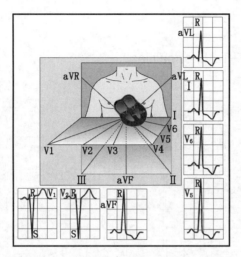

图6-1　左心室肥大中QRS波电压改变

Fig. 6-1　QRS voltages changes in left ventricular hypertrophy

amplitude in leads opposite to the left ventricle wall (V1 and V2) (see Fig. 6-1). Limb lead voltage criteria include R wave amplitude > 1.5 mV in lead Ⅰ, > 1.1 mV in lead aVL, > 2.0 mV in lead aVF, and the sum of $R_Ⅰ + S_Ⅲ > 2.5$ mV. Precordial lead voltage criteria include R wave amplitude > 2.5 mV in leads V5 or V6, the sum of $R_{V5\ or\ V6} + S_{V1}$ > 3.5 mV. More recently, the sum of $S_{V3} + R_{aVL}$ > 2.8 mV for male and > 2.0 mV for female, referred to as the "Cornell voltage," has been used for diagnosis. For measurements of QRS voltages, see Fig. 6-2.

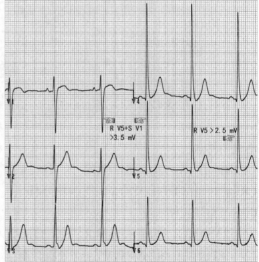

图6-2　QRS波电压的测量

Fig. 6-2　Measurements of QRS voltages

图例7 左心室肥大，ST-T改变

Case 7 Left Ventricular Hypertrophy, ST-T Abnormalities

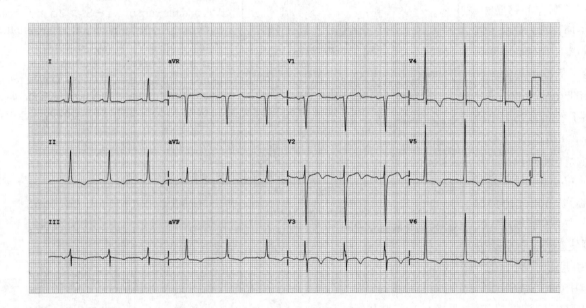

心电图特点

1. 心 率: 73次/min; PR间 期: 168 ms; QRS波时间: 94 ms; QT/QTc间期: 412/454 ms; QRS波电轴: 39°。

2. V5导联R波振幅>2.5 mV, R_{V5}+S_{V1}>3.5 mV。

3. T波在 Ⅰ、Ⅱ、aVF和V3 ~ V6导联倒置。

4. V5和V6导联ST段压低 ≥ 0.05 mV。

ECG Characteristics

1. HR: 73 bpm; PR: 168 ms; QRS D: 94 ms; QT/QTc: 412/454 ms; QRS axis: 39°.

2. R wave amplitude in lead V5 is > 2.5 mV, R_{V5} + S_{V1} > 3.5 mV.

3. T waves are inverted in leads Ⅰ, Ⅱ, aVF and V3 ~ V6.

4. ST segments depression in leads V5 and V6 is ≥ 0.05 mV.

ECG Interpretation

Sinus rhythm, left ventricular hypertrophy, ST-T abnormalities
The non-voltage criteria for left ventricular hypertrophy include

心电图诊断与解析

诊断: 窦性心律; 左心室肥大; ST-T改变。

解析: 用于诊断左心室肥大的非电压标准包括: ST-T改变、QRS波增宽、电轴左偏、左房异常和QT间期延长。ST-T改变表现为J点压低和下斜型ST段压低, 并伴有T波倒置。根据"AHA/ACC/HRS建议", 应用"继发性ST-T改变"这一术语取代"劳损"和"典型劳损"等曾用术语[1]。左心室壁增厚和激动时间延长, 可导致QRS波增宽。电轴左偏和P波异常只用于辅助诊断。此心电图T波改变的识别参见图7-1。

ST-T abnormalities, prolonged QRS duration, left axis deviation, left atrial abnormalities and prolonged QT interval. The ST-T abnormalities consist of J-point depression, down-sloping depression of the ST segment, and inversion of the T wave. According to "AHA/ACCF/HRS Recommendations", the term "secondary ST-T abnormalities" is preferred over the terms "strain" and "typical strain" to be used[1]. The increase in the thickness of the left ventricular wall prolongs the ventricular activation time and may result in lengthening the total QRS duration. Left axis deviation and P-wave abnormalities should only be used as a supporting criterion. For T wave abnormalities in this ECG, see Fig. 7-1.

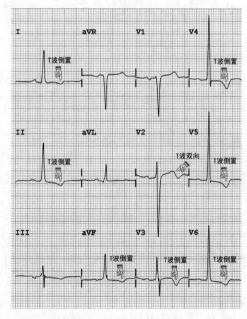

图7-1 T波改变

Fig. 7-1 T wave abnormalities

图例8 右心室肥大

Case 8 Right Ventricular Hypertrophy

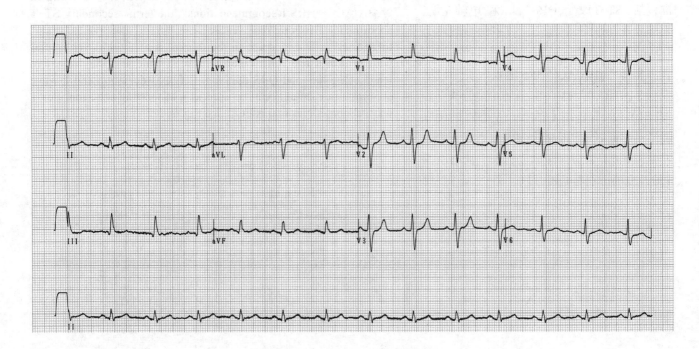

心电图特点

1. 心率：81次/min；PR间期：146 ms；QRS波时间：102 ms；QT/QTc间期：374/434 ms；QRS波电轴：122°。

2. V1导联单向高大R波，aVR导联R/Q>1。$R_{V1}+S_{V5}>1.05$ mV。电轴右偏>90°。

ECG Characteristics

1. HR: 81 bpm; PR: 146 ms; QRS D: 102 ms; QT/QTc: 374/434 ms; QRS axis: 122°.

2. The tall R wave is in lead V1, R/Q ratio in lead aVR is > 1. $R_{V1}+S_{V5}>1.05$ mV. Right axis deviation is > 90°.

ECG Interpretation

Sinus rhythm, right ventricular hypertrophy.

心电图诊断与解析

诊断：窦性心律；右心室肥大。

解析：正常心脏，左心室电势占优势。右心室肥大需要达到一定程度才能逆转优势，出现心电图改变。因此心电图诊断右心室肥大并不敏感。轻度右心室肥大，心电图可以正常。重度肥大，心电图逆转为右心室占优势。右心室所产生的电势向右向前。V1导联位置面对右心室壁，因此在V1导联形成高大R波。在肢体导联上向右的电势增加，表现为电轴右偏。根据"AHA/ACC/HRS建议"[1]，电轴右偏和右胸导联上前向电势，是心电图诊断右心室肥大的必需条件，见图8-1。

The force of left ventricular activation dominates the balance in a normal heart, which requires usually a considerable degree of right ventricular hypertrophy to shift the balance and to be reflected on the ECG. Thus the ECG is relatively insensitive to right ventricular hypertrophy, and may be normal in mild cases. With severe hypertrophy, the force of right ventricular depolarization may dominate on the ECG. The forces generated by right ventricular depolarization are directed rightwards and anteriorly. Lead V1 lies closest to the right ventricular wall and records the tall R wave . The limb leads show right axis deviation under increased rightward force.

According to "AHA/ACCF/HRS Recommendations", right axis deviation and prominent anterior forces in the right precordial leads should be required for the ECG diagnosis of RVH in nearly all cases,[1] see Fig. 8-1.

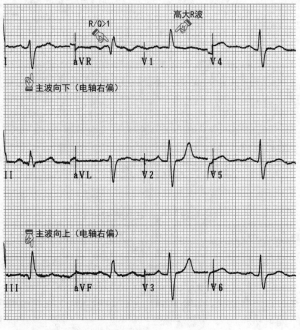

图8-1　高大R波和电轴右偏

Fig. 8-1　Tall R wave and right axis deviation

图例9　右心室肥大,ST-T改变

Case 9　Right Ventricular Hypertrophy, ST-T Abnormalities

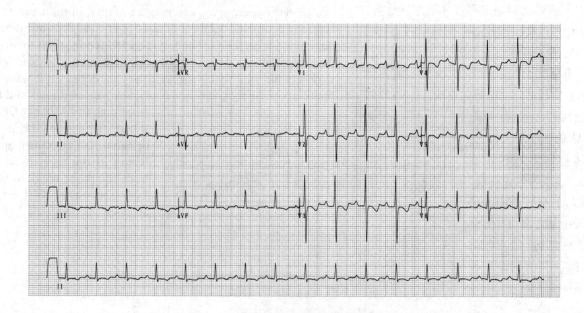

心电图特点

1. 心率: 97次/min, PR间期: 200 ms; QRS波时间: 78 ms; QT/QTc间期: 376/477 ms; QRS波电轴: 112°。

2. V1导联单向高大R波, V5导联R/S=1。$R_{V1}+S_{V5} > 1.05$ mV。电轴右偏 > 90°。T波在Ⅱ、Ⅲ、aVF和V1 ~ V5导联倒置, V6导联低平。V2 ~ V4导联ST段压低 > 0.05 mV。

ECG Characteristics

1. HR: 97 bpm; PR: 200 ms; QRS D: 78 ms; QT/QTc: 376/477 ms; QRS axis: 112°.

2. The tall R wave is in lead V1, R/S ratio in lead V5 is=1. $R_{V1} + S_{V5} > 1.05$ mV. Right axis deviation is > 90°. T waves are inverted in leads Ⅱ, Ⅲ, aVF and V1~V5, low and flat in lead V6. ST segments depression in leads V2 ~ V4 is > 0.05 mV.

ECG Interpretation

Sinus rhythm, right ventricular hypertrophy, ST-T abnormalities.

心电图诊断与解析

诊断：窦性心律；右心室肥大；ST-T改变。

解析：右心室肥大所见的ST-T改变通常位于右胸导联（V1和V2导联），包括ST段压低和T波倒置。根据"AHA/ACC/HRS建议"：建议用"继发性ST-T改变"术语，而不是"劳损"术语[1]。此心电图中ST-T改变累及至左胸导联（V4～V6），显著的改变是T波倒置（见图9-1），提示可能伴有原发性ST-T改变，详见后文（图例17）。

For right ventricular hypertrophy, ST-T abnormalities are usually observed in the right precordial leads (V1 and V2). The ST-T abnormalities include ST segment depression and T wave inversion. According to "AHA/ACCF/HRS Recommendations", these ST-T abnormalities are better referred to as "secondary ST-T abnormality" than as "strain"[1]. In this ECG, the ST-T abnormalities extended to the left precordial leads (V4~V6). The remarkable change of T wave inversion (see Fig. 9-1) suggests possible primary ST-T abnormalities coexistence, more details in following article (case 17).

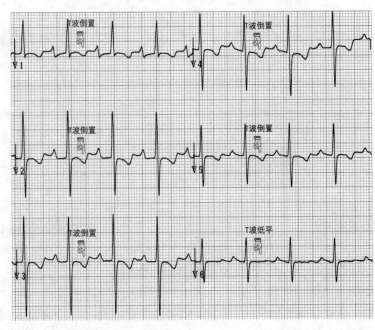

图9-1　T波改变

Fig. 9-1　T wave abnormalities

图例 10　右心房肥大，右心室肥大

Case 10　Right Atrial Enlargement, Right Ventricular Hypertrophy

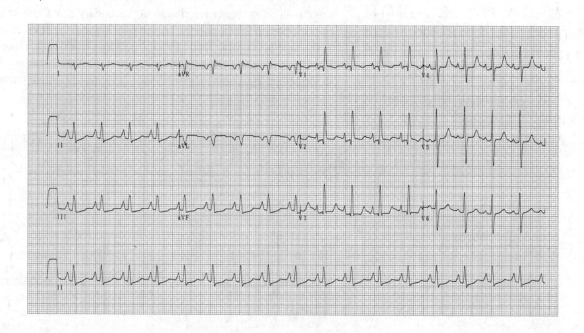

心电图特点

1. 心率：105次/min；PR间期：140 ms；QRS波时间：110 ms；QT/QTc间期：368/486 ms；QRS波电轴：101°。

2. P波在 I 和 II 导联直立，在 aVR 导联倒置；心率 > 100次/min。

3. II、III 和 aVF 导联 P 波振幅 > 0.25 mV。

ECG Characteristics

1. HR: 105 bpm; PR: 140 ms; QRS D: 110 ms; QT/QTc: 368/486 ms; QRS axis: 101°.

2. P waves are upright in leads I and II, and inverted in lead aVR; HR is > 100 bpm.

3. P waves amplitude is > 0.25 mV in lead II, III and aVF.

4. The tall R wave in lead V1, $R_{V1} + S_{V5} > 1.05$ mV.

5. Right axis deviation is > 90°.

4. V1 导联单向高大 R 波，$R_{V1}+S_{V5} > 1.05\,mV$。

5. 电轴右偏 > 90°。

心电图诊断与解析

诊断：窦性心动过速；右心房肥大；右心室肥大；T 波改变。

解析：临床上，右心室肥大大部分伴有右心房肥大，如先天性心脏病、慢性阻塞性肺病和肺动脉高压。此心电图是一例先天性心脏病患者，心电图改变提示右心室肥大伴右心房肥大，可有助于临床疾病评定。右心室肥大伴右心房肥大的心电图改变见图 10-1。

ECG Interpretation

Sinus tachycardia, right atrial enlargement, right ventricular hypertrophy, t wave abnormalities.

In cases such as congenital heart disease, chronic obstructive pulmonary disease and pulmonary hypertension, right ventricular hypertrophy is often combined with right atrial enlargement. This ECG is an example of a case with congenital heart disease. The ECG changes suggest right atrial enlargement and right ventricular hypertrophy, which may provide information for the patient's clinical assessment. See Fig. 10-1 for the ECG changes.

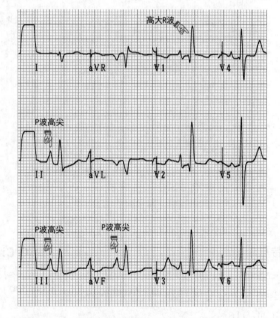

图 10-1　右心室肥大伴右心房肥大的心电图改变

Fig. 10-1　ECG changes in right atrial enlargement and right ventricular hypertrophy

图例11　左心房肥大,右心室肥大

Case 11　Left Atrial Enlargement, Right Ventricular Hypertrophy

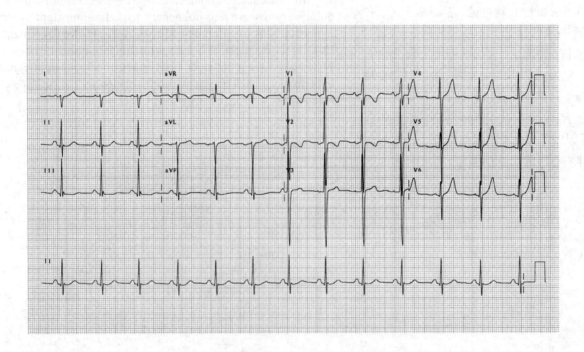

心电图特点

1. 心率: 77次/min; PR间期: 162 ms; QRS波时间: 95 ms; QT/QTc间期: 359/406 ms; QRS波电轴: 116°。

2. P波时间 > 120 ms, V1导联Ptf绝对值 > 0.04 mm·s。V1导联单向高大R波,

ECG Characteristics

1. HR: 77 bpm; PR: 162 ms; QRS D: 95 ms; QT/QTc: 359/406 ms; QRS axis: 116°.

2. P wave duration is > 120 ms, P-terminal force in lead V1 is > 0.04 mm·s. The tall R wave is in lead V1, R/Q ratio in lead aVR is > 1, R/S ratio in lead V5 is < 1. $R_{V1} + S_{V5}$ > 1.05 mV. Right axis deviation is > 90°.

aVR 导联 R/Q > 1，V5 导联 R/S<1。$R_{V1}+S_{V5}$ > 1.05 mV。电轴右偏 > 90°。

心电图诊断与解析

诊断：窦性心律；左心房肥大；右心室肥大；T波改变。

解析：临床上，左心房肥大伴右心室肥大最常见于二尖瓣病变。此心电图见于一例风湿性心脏病二尖瓣狭窄的患者，心电图改变提示左心房肥大伴右心室肥大，可有助于临床疾病评定，见图11-1。

ECG Interpretation

Sinus rhythm, left atrial enlargement, right ventricular hypertrophy, T wave abnormalities.

Clinically, most cases of left atrial enlargement with right ventricular hypertrophy indicate mitral valvular diseases. This ECG is an example of a case with rheumatic mitral stenosis. The ECG changes suggest left atrial enlargement and right ventricular hypertrophy, which may provide information for the patient's clinical assessment. See Fig. 11-1.

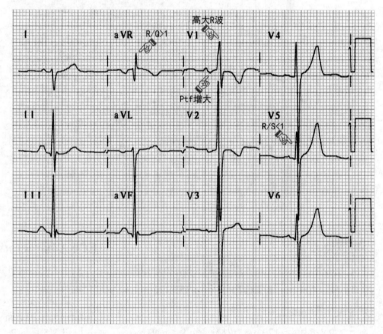

图 11-1　左心房肥大伴右心室肥大的心电图改变

Fig. 11-1　ECG changes in left atrial enlargement and right ventricular hypertrophy

图例12　左心房肥大，左心室肥大

Case 12　Left Atrial Enlargement, Left Ventricular Hypertrophy

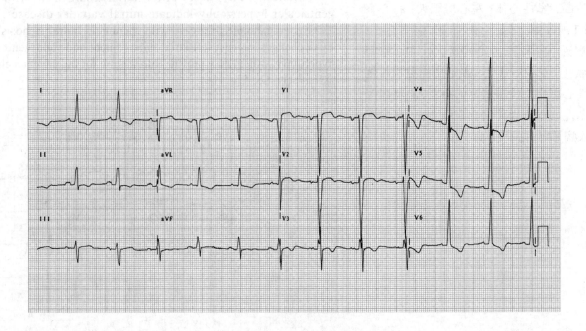

心电图特点

1. 心率: 72次/min; PR间期: 191 ms; QRS波时间: 104 ms; QT/QTc间期: 357/391 ms; QRS波电轴: 13°。

2. P波时间>120 ms, 双峰, 峰间距>40 ms, V1导联Ptf绝对值>0.04 mm·s。V5导联R波振幅>2.5 mV, $R_{V5}+S_{V1}$>3.5 mV。QRS波增

ECG Characteristics

1. HR: 72 bpm; PR: 191 ms; QRS D: 104 ms; QT/QTc: 357/391 ms; QRS axis: 13°.

2. P wave duration is > 120 ms, notched with the inter-peak duration > 40 ms, P-terminal force in lead V1 is > 0.04 mm·s. R wave in lead V5 is > 2.5 mV, $R_{V5} + S_{V1}$ > 3.5 mV. QRS duration is >100 ms. T waves are inverted in leads Ⅰ, Ⅱ, aVL and V3~V6. ST segment depression in leads V4 ~ V6 > 0.05 mV.

宽 > 100 ms。T波在Ⅰ、Ⅱ、aVL和V3 ~ V6导联倒置。V4 ~ V6导联ST段压低 > 0.05 mV。

心电图诊断与解析

诊断：窦性心律；左心房肥大；左心室肥大；ST-T改变。

解析：临床上，左心室肥大伴左心房肥大常见于高血压心脏病、瓣膜性心脏病和心肌病。此心电图见于一例长期高血压患者，心电图改变提示左心室肥大伴左心房肥大，可有助于临床评定高血压对心脏的损害。左心室肥大伴左心房肥大的心电图改变见图12-1。

ECG Interpretation

Sinus rhythm, left atrial enlargement, left ventricular hypertrophy, ST-T abnormalities.

Clinically, left ventricular hypertrophy with left atrial enlargement is most common in hypertensive heart disease, valvular heart disease and cardiomyopathy. This ECG is an example of a case with long-term hypertension. The ECG changes suggesting left ventricular hypertrophy with left atrial enlargement (see Fig. 12-1) may help to evaluate cardiac damage by hypertension.

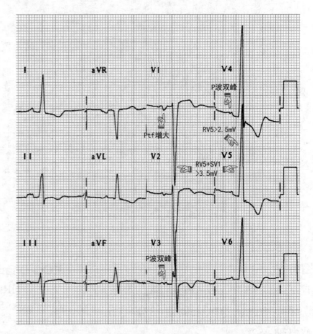

图 12-1 左心室肥大伴左心房肥大的心电图改变

Fig. 12-1 ECG changes in left atrial enlargement and left ventricular hypertrophy

图例 13　双心室肥大

Case 13　Biventricular Hypertrophy

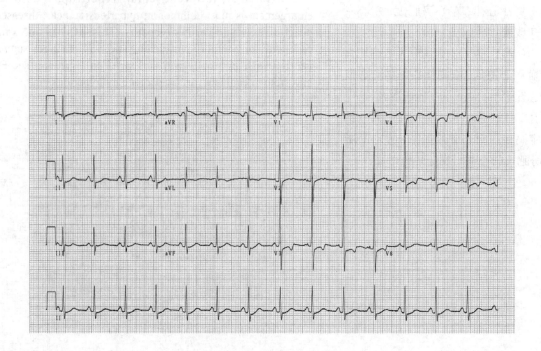

心电图特点

1. 心率：85次/min；PR间期：148 ms；QRS波时间：86 ms；QT/QTc间期：374/445 ms；QRS波电轴：52°。

2. V5导联R波振幅 > 2.5 mV，$R_{V5}+S_{V1}$ > 3.5 mV，V1导联高大R波。V4导联R波和S

ECG Characteristics

1. HR: 85 bpm; PR: 148 ms; QRS D: 86 ms; QT/QTc: 374/445 ms; QRS axis: 52°.

2. R wave in lead V5 is > 2.5 mV, R_{V5} + S_{V1} > 3.5 mV, the tall R wave in lead V1.

3. The R wave combined S wave is close to 6.0 mV in lead V4.

4. T waves are inverted in leads V3 ~ V5, low and flat in lead V6.

波振幅之和近似于6.0 mV。T波在V3 ~ V5
导联倒置，在V6导联低平。V3 ~ V6导联ST
段压低≥0.05 mV。

心电图诊断与解析

诊断：窦性心律；双心室肥大；ST-T改变。

解析：临床上，许多心脏疾病可以引起
双心室肥大。由于左右心室电势的相互抵
消，心电图对双心室的诊断不
敏感性。根据"AHA/ACC/
HRS建议"：左心室肥大若伴
有V5或V6导联S波增大、电
轴右偏、一些导联上QRS波
呈R/S型和右心房异常，则提
示同时存在右心室肥大。先
天性心脏病有右心室肥大，
若伴有V2 ~ V4导联QRS波
呈R/S型，R波和S波振幅之
和＞6.0 mV，提示同时存在左
心室肥大[1]。此心电图见于
一例肥厚性心肌病的患者，心
电图特点是V5导联R波振幅
显著增高伴V1导联高大R波，
V4导联R波和S波振幅之和
近似于6.0 mV，提示双心室肥
大（见图13-1）。

5. ST segments depression in leads V3 ~ V6 is ≥ 0.05 mV.

ECG Interpretation

Sinus rhythm, biventricular hypertrophy, ST-T abnormalities.

Clinically, various heart diseases can cause hypertrophy both in right and left ventricles. Because of the cancellation of increased forces from both ventricles, ECG is particularly insensitive to biventricular hypertrophy. According to "AHA/ACCF/HRS Recommendations":"In the presence of ECG criteria for left ventricular hypertrophy, the presence of prominent S waves in V5 or V6, right axis deviation, unusually tall biphasic R/S complexes in several leads, and signs of right atrial abnormality are useful signs that right ventricular hypertrophy may also be present. In patients with congenital heart defects and right ventricular hypertrophy, the presence of combined tall R waves and deep S waves in leads V2 to V4, with combined amplitude greater than 60 mm (6.0 mV), suggests the presence of left ventricular hypertrophy."[1] This ECG is an example of a case with hypertrophic cardiomyopathy. The amplitude of R wave in lead V5 is significantly increased and the tall R wave in lead V1 is observed. The amplitude sum of R and S wave in lead V4 is close to 6.0 mV. All of these ECG changes (see Fig. 13-1) suggest biventricular hypertrophy.

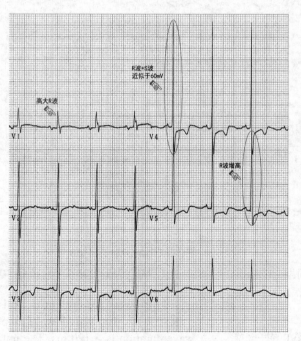

图13-1 双心室肥大的心电图改变

Fig. 13-1　ECG changes in biventricular hypertrophy

图例14 双心房肥大

Case 14 Bi-atrial Enlargement

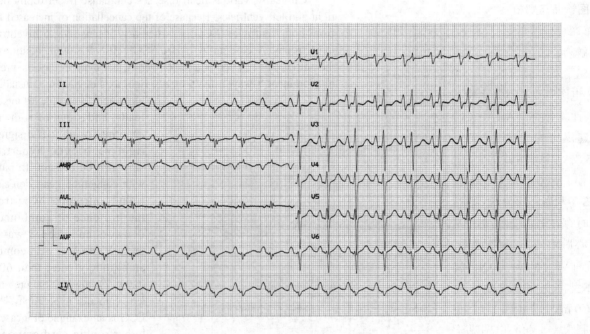

心电图特点

1. 心率：102次/min；PR间期：178 ms；QRS波时间：104 ms；QT/QTc间期：362/473 ms；QRS波电轴：−65°。

2. P波在Ⅰ和Ⅱ导联直立，在aVR导联倒置；心率>100次/min。Ⅱ导联P波振幅>0.25 mV；P波时间>120 ms。V1导联P波初始正向>0.15 mV，

ECG Characteristics

1. HR: 102 bpm; PR: 178 ms; QRS D: 104 ms; QT/QTc: 362/473 ms; QRS axis: −65°.

2. P waves are upright in leads Ⅰ and Ⅱ, and inverted in lead aVR; HR is > 100 bpm. P wave amplitude is > 0.25 mV in lead Ⅱ; P wave duration is > 120 ms. The initial positive deflection of P wave is > 0.15 mV and the terminal negative deflection of P wave is > 0.04 mm·s in lead V1.

终末负向>0.04mm·s。

3. 6个肢体导联QRS波振幅均<0.5 mV。V4～V6导联QRS波呈rS型。

心电图诊断与解析

诊断：窦性心动过速；双心房肥大（异常）；肢体导联低电压；电轴右偏；顺钟向转位。

解析：心电图上双心房肥大的特点是同时具有左右心房肥大的改变，P波振幅增加和时间延长，V1导联高大双相，起始波和终末波均增加。几十年来，沿用"双心房肥大"这一术语来描述这一现象。新近，根据"AHA/ACC/HRS建议"，P波异常应用"心房异常"诊断，而不用"心房扩大""负荷过重""劳损或肥厚"等术语[1]。国内尚未确定相关术语。临床上，双心房肥大或双心房异常并不常见。此心电图见于一例限制性心肌病的患者：首先，Ⅱ导联P波振幅 > 0.25 mV，P波增宽 > 120 ms；其次是V1导联P波，初始正向 > 0.15 mV，终末负向 > 0.04 mm，双向振幅均增加（见图14-1）。所有这些心电图改变提示双心房肥大（异常）。

3. QRS amplitudes in all six limb leads are <0.5 mV. QRS complexes represent rS pattern in leads V4 ~ V6.

ECG Interpretation

Sinus tachycardia, bi-atrial enlargement (combined atrial abnormality), low voltage in limb leads, right axis deviation, clockwise rotation.

The bi-atrial abnormality is indicated by the presence of the features of both right and left atrial abnormalities: tall and widened P wave, biphasic in lead V1, increasing in both initial positive and terminal negative deflection in lead V1. The term "Bi-atrial enlargement" has been used to describe the situation for several decades. Recently, according to "AHA/ACCF/HRS Recommendations", "abnormal P waves should usually be referred to as right or left 'atrial abnormality' rather than enlargement, overload, strain, or hypertrophy."[1] The term is not yet to be determined in China. Bi-atrial enlargement or combined atrial abnormality is not very common clinically. This ECG is an example of a case with restrictive cardiomyopathy. First, the amplitude of P wave is > 0.25 mV in lead Ⅱ and the duration of P wave is > 120 ms. Second, P wave in lead V1, initial deflection is greater than 0.15 mV and terminal deflection is greater than 0.04 mm·s, both amplitudes increase (see Fig. 14-1). All of these ECG changes suggest bi-atrial enlargement or combined atrial abnormality.

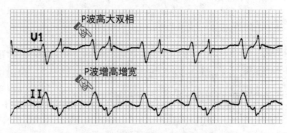

图14-1 双心房肥大的心电图改变

Fig. 14-1 ECG changes in bi-atrial enlargement

图例15　T波改变

Case 15　T Wave Abnormalities

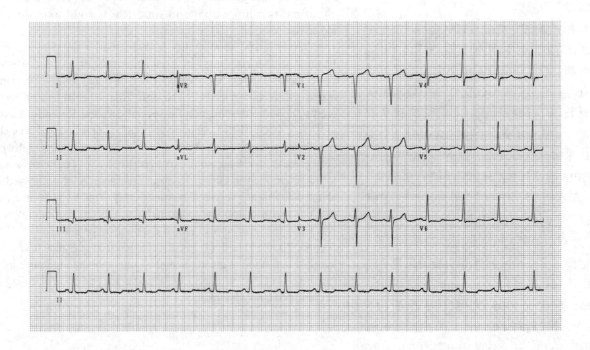

心电图特点

1. 心率：82次/min；PR间期：142 ms；QRS波时间：94 ms；QT/QTc间期：384/448 ms；QRS波电轴：49°。

2. T波在Ⅰ、Ⅱ、aVF和V4~V6导联低平。

3. V5和V6导联ST段压低<0.05 mV。

ECG Characteristics

1. HR: 82 bpm; PR: 142 ms; QRS D: 94 ms; QT/QTc: 384/448 ms; QRS axis: 49°.

2. T waves are low and flat in leads Ⅰ, Ⅱ, aVF and V4 ~ V6.

3. ST segments depression in leads V5 and V6 is < 0.05 mV.

ECG Interpretation

Sinus rhythm, T wave abnormalities.

心电图诊断与解析

诊断：窦性心律；T波改变。

解析：T波改变可伴或不伴ST段改变。根据"AHA/ACC/HRS建议"，关于T波正常与否的概念是："1月以上的儿童，V1～V3导联T波常倒置。12～20岁青少年，aVF导联T波可轻微倒置，V2导联T波可倒置。20岁以上成人，aVR导联T波倒置，aVL、Ⅲ和V1导联T波可直立或倒置。Ⅰ、Ⅱ和V3～V6导联T波直立"[2]，高尖、双向、低平和倒置是描写T波改变的一些术语。若T波振幅<同导联R波振幅的1/10，则称为T波低平。此心电图上T波改变的识别见图15-1。

T wave abnormality can occur in the presence or absence of ST segment abnormality. According to "AHA/ACCF/HRS Recommendations", the conception of normal or abnormal T wave is that: "In children older than 1 month, the T wave is often inverted in leads V1, V2, and V3. In adolescents 12 years old and older and in young adults less than 20 years of age, the T wave may be slightly inverted in aVF and inverted in lead V2. In adults 20 years old and older, the normal T wave is inverted in aVR; upright or inverted in leads aVL, Ⅲ, and V1; and upright in leads Ⅰ and Ⅱ and in chest leads V3 through V6."[2] Several terms such as "peaked," "biphasic," "low" and "inverted" are being used to describe the T wave abnormality. The T wave is considered low when its amplitude is < 10% of the amplitude of R wave in the same lead. For T wave abnormalities in this ECG, see Fig. 15-1.

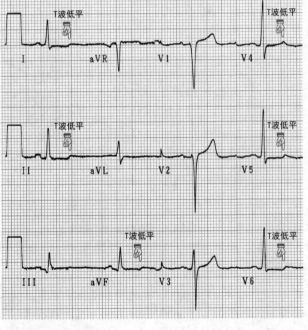

图15-1 T波改变

Fig. 15-1 T wave abnormalities

图例16 T波改变

Case 16 T Wave Abnormalities

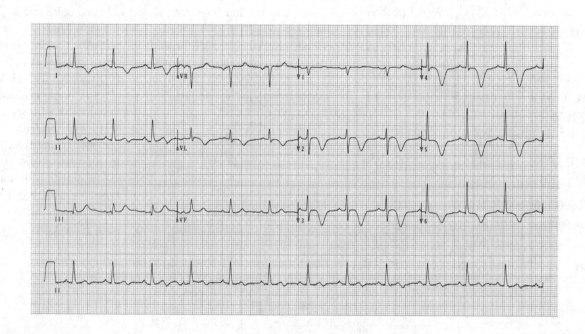

心电图特点

1. 心率：75次/min；PR间期：152 ms；QRS波时间：88 ms；QT/QTc间期：464/518 ms；QRS波电轴：40°。

2. T波在 I 、aVL 和V2 ~ V6导联倒置或深倒置，在 II 导联正负双向。V5和V6导联ST段压低<0.05 mV。

ECG Characteristics

1. HR: 75 bpm; PR: 152 ms; QRS D: 88 ms; QT/QTc: 464/518 ms; QRS axis: 40°.

2. T waves are inverted or deep inverted in leads I , aVL and V2 ~ V6, and biphasic in lead II . ST segment depression in leads V5 and V6 is < 0.05 mV.

ECG Interpretation

Sinus rhythm, T wave abnormalities, QT interval prolonged.

心电图诊断与解析

诊断: 窦性心律; T波改变; QT间期延长。

解析: 根据"AHA/ACC/HRS建议": "Ⅰ、Ⅱ、aVL和V2~V6导联T波振幅-0.1~-0.5 mV定义为T波倒置; -0.5~-1.0 mV为T波深倒置; >-1.0 mV为巨大倒置T波。T波振幅低于同导联R波振幅的1/10为T波低平; T波平坦是指Ⅰ、Ⅱ、aVL和V4~V6导联, T波振幅在0.1~-0.1 mV, 其中Ⅰ、Ⅱ、aVL导联R波振幅>0.3 mV"[2]。临床上, 评定T波改变, 侧壁V5和V6最为重要。此心电图T波改变的识别见图16-1。

According to "AHA/ACCF/HRS Recommendations", "As more quantitative descriptors, it is proposed that the T wave in leads Ⅰ, Ⅱ, aVL, and V2 to V6 be reported as inverted when the T-wave amplitude is from −0.1 to −0.5 mV, as deep negative when the amplitude is from −0.5 to−1.0 mV, and as giant negative when the amplitude is less than−1.0 mV. In addition, the T wave may be called low when its amplitude is less than 10% of the R-wave amplitude in the same lead and as flat when the peak T-wave amplitude is between 0.1 and−0.1 mV in leads Ⅰ, Ⅱ, aVL (with an R wave taller than 0.3 mV), and V4 to V6."[2] Clinically, negative T waves in lateral precordial leads V5 and V6 is particularly important in evaluations of T wave abnormalities. For T wave abnormalities in this ECG, see Fig. 16-1.

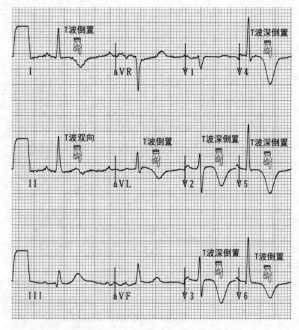

图 16-1 T波改变

Fig. 16-1 T wave abnormalities

图例17 ST段改变

Case 17 ST Segment Abnormalities

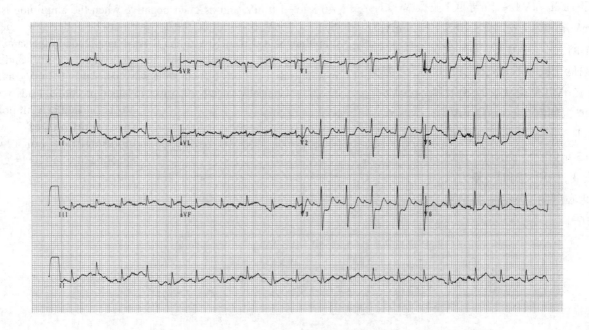

心电图特点

1. 心率：116次/min；PR间期：148 ms；QRS波时间：84 ms；QT/QTc间期：334/464 ms；QRS波电轴：74°。

2. V2～V5导联ST段压低＞0.05 mV，Ⅲ和aVF导联抬高＞0.1 mV。

ECG Characteristics

1. HR: 116 bpm; PR: 148 ms; QRS D: 84 ms; QT/QTc: 334/464 ms; QRS axis: 74°.

2. ST segments depression in leads V2 ~ V5 is > 0.05 mV, elevation in leads Ⅲ and aVF is > 0.1 mV.

ECG Interpretation

Sinus tachycardia, ST segment abnormalities.

According to "AHA/ACCF/HRS Recommendations", the

心电图诊断与解析

诊断：窦性心动过速；ST段改变。

解析：根据"AHA/ACC/HRS建议"，ST-T改变的概念包括："原发性ST-T改变是由跨膜动作电位复极部分的形态和（或）时程异常引起的，除极是正常的"，而"继发性ST-T改变是由心室除极顺序和（或）时程异常所致，心电图表现为QRS波形态或时限异常"[2]。原发性异常可见于多种临床情况，如心肌缺血、心肌炎、中毒和电解质紊乱。ST段改变可以描述为抬高（上移）和压低（下移）。ST段抬高可进一步描述为弓背向上或凹面向上，而ST段压低可进一步描述为水平型、下斜型和上斜型。此心电图ST段改变的识别见图17-1。

conception of ST-T abnormalities include:"Abnormalities in the ST segment and T wave, which are the result of changes in the shape and/or duration of the repolarization phases of the transmembrane action potential and occur in the absence of changes in depolarization, are referred to as primary repolarization abnormalities", "Abnormalities in the ST segment and T wave that occur as the direct result of changes in the sequence and/or duration of ventricular depolarization, manifested electrocardiographically as changes in QRS shape and/or duration, are referred to as secondary repolarization abnormalities."[2]

The primary abnormalities may be caused by a variety of events, including ischemia, myocarditis, drugs, toxins, and electrolyte abnormalities. The ST segment can be described as "elevated" and "depressed". The elevated ST segment may be further characterized as "convex upwards" or "concave upwards", and the depressed ST segment may be further characterized as "horizontal" "downsloping", or "upsloping". For ST segment abnormalities in ECG, see Fig. 17-1.

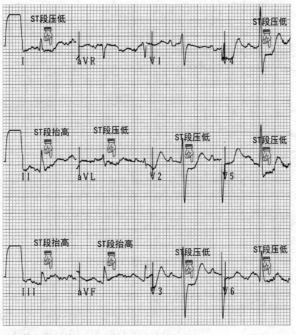

图 17-1 ST段改变

Fig. 17-1 ST segment abnormalities

图例18 ST段改变

Case 18 ST Segment Abnormalities

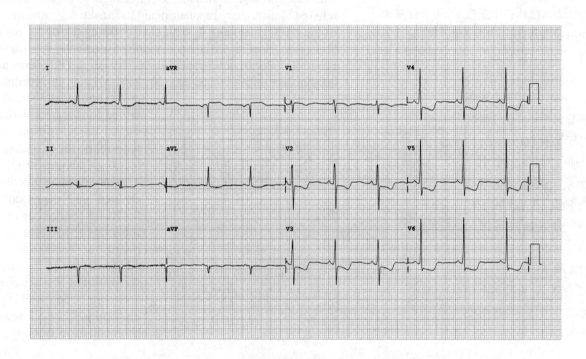

心电图特点

1. 心率: 68次/min; PR间期: 132 ms; QRS波时间: 80 ms; QT/QTc间期: 392/417 ms; QRS波电轴: −30°。

2. Ⅰ、aVL 和 V2 ~ V6 导联 ST 段压低 > 0.05 mV。T波在 Ⅰ 和 aVL 导联低平, 在 V2 ~

ECG Characteristics

1. HR: 68 bpm; PR: 132 ms; QRS D: 80 ms; QT/QTc: 392/417 ms; QRS axis: −30°.

2. ST segments depression in leads Ⅰ, aVL and V2 ~ V6 is > 0.05 mV.T waves are low and flat in leads Ⅰ and aVL, biphasic in leads V2 ~ V6.

V6导联负正双向。

心电图诊断与解析

诊断：窦性心律；ST–T改变。

解析：ST段改变可伴或不伴T波改变。此心电图ST段改变伴发T波改变。V2～V6导联中，ST段下斜型压低和T波负正双向是此心电图的特点，见图18–1。ST段移位（抬高或压低）最常用于心电图诊断心肌缺血或心肌梗死，下斜型或水平型ST段压低，提示可能存在心肌缺血。

ECG Interpretation

Sinus rhythm, ST–T abnormalities.

ST segment abnormalities can occur with or without T wave abnormalities. This ECG shows ST segment abnormalities combined with T wave abnormalities. The features of this ECG are downsloping ST segment depression and biphasic T wave in leads V2 ～ V6, see Fig. 18–1. Deviation (elevation or depression) of the ST segment from the baseline is the most common clinical use of ECG for diagnosis of ischemia or infarction. Downsloping or horizontal ST segment depression may indicate ischemia.

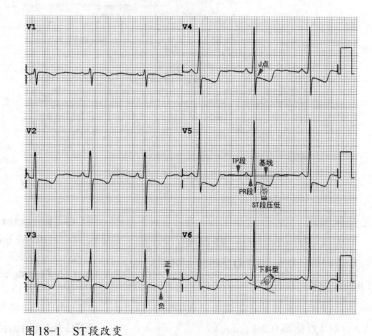

图 18–1 ST段改变

Fig. 18–1 ST segment abnormalities

图例 19　ST-T 改变

Case 19　ST-T Abnormalities

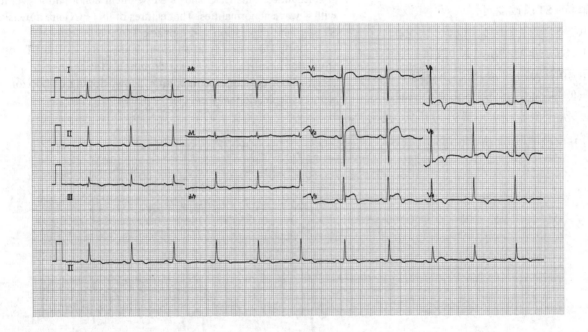

心电图特点

1. 心率：67 次/min；PR 间期：165 ms；QRS 波时间：92 ms；QT/QTc 间期：391/413 ms；QRS 波电轴：60°。

2. Ⅱ和 V4 导联 J 点抬高 > 0.1 mV，V1 ~ V3 导联 J 点抬高 0.2 ~ 0.3 mV。

3. T 波在Ⅱ、Ⅲ、aVF 和 V2 ~ V4 导联倒置。

ECG Characteristics

1. HR: 67 bpm; PR: 165 ms; QRS D: 92 ms; QT/QTc: 391/413 ms; QRS axis: 60°.

2. J points elevation in leads Ⅱ and V4 is > 0.1 mV, in leads V1 ~ V3 is 0.2 ~ 0.3 mV.

3. T waves are inverted in leads Ⅱ, Ⅲ, aVF and V2 ~ V4.

ECG Interpretation

Sinus rhythm, ST-T abnormalities.

心电图诊断与解析

诊断：窦性心律；ST-T改变。

解析：正常人群，V1～V3导联可见ST段抬高，通常V2导联最为显著。根据"AHA/ACC/HRS建议"：40岁及以上男性，V2和V3导联J点抬高不应超过0.2 mV，其他导联不应超过0.1 mV；40岁以下男性，V2和V3导联J点抬高不超过0.25 mV；女性V2和V3导联J点抬高不应超过0.15 mV，其他导联不应超过0.1 mV[3]。评定ST段抬高主要关注急性心肌梗死中的心肌缺血或损失，详见后文（图例20）。此心电图ST-T改变的识别见图19-1。

ST segment elevation in leads V1 ~ V3 may occur in normal group, and is usually most pronounced in lead V2. According to "AHA/ACCF/HRS Recommendations", "For men 40 years of age and older, the threshold value for abnormal J-point elevation should be 0.2 mV in leads V2 and V3 and 0.1 mV in all other leads. For men less than 40 years of age, the value should be 0.25 mV in leads V2 and V3. For women, the threshold value should be 0.15 mV in leads V2 and V3 and greater than 0.1 mV in all other leads."[3] Evaluation ST segment elevation is particular concern of myocardial ischemia or injurious in acute myocardial infarction, as discussed in detail in the following article (case 20). For ST-T abnormalities in this ECG, see Fig. 19-1.

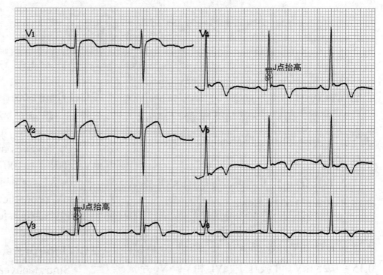

图 19-1　ST-T改变

Fig. 19-1　ST-T abnormalities

图例20　急性广泛前壁心肌梗死（早期）

Case 20　Acute Extensive Anterior Myocardial Infarction (Early Stage)

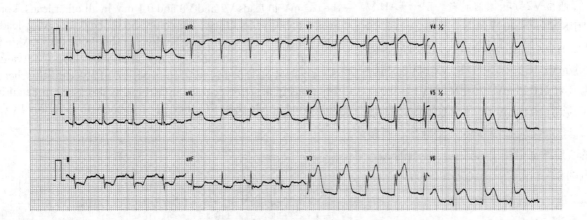

心电图特点

　　1. 心率：102次/min；PR间期：145 ms；QRS波时间：82 ms；QT/QTc间期：320/420 ms；QRS波电轴：6°。

　　2. P波在Ⅰ和Ⅱ导联直立，在aVR导联倒置；心率 > 100次/min。

　　3. Ⅰ、aVL和V2 ~ V6导联ST段抬高0.25 ~ 1.35 mV，Ⅲ和aVF导联ST段压低0.15 ~ 0.25 mV。T波在Ⅰ、aVL和V1 ~ V6导联直立高耸。所有导联未见异常Q波。

心电图诊断与解析

　　诊断：窦性心动过速；急性广泛前壁心

ECG Characteristics

　　1. HR: 102 bpm; PR: 145 ms; QRS D: 82 ms; QT/QTc: 320/420 ms; QRS axis: 6°.

　　2. P waves are upright in leads Ⅰ and Ⅱ, and inverted in lead aVR; HR is > 100 bpm.

　　3. ST segments elevation in leads Ⅰ, aVL and V2 ~ V6 is 0.25 ~ 1.35 mV, depression in leads Ⅲ and aVF is 0.15 ~ 0.25 mV. T waves are tall and peaked in leads Ⅰ, aVL and V2 ~ V6. There is no pathological Q wave in all leads.

ECG Interpretation

　　Sinus tachycardia, acute extensive anterior myocardial infarction (early stage).

　　When myocardial blood supply is abruptly reduced or occluded for a region of heart, a sequence of events occur beginning with ischemia,

肌梗死（早期）。

解析：当部分心肌血流突然减少或阻断，将出现心肌缺血、损伤和坏死等一系列改变，这一事件即为心肌梗死。根据"AHA/ACC/HRS建议"，"急性心肌缺血和梗死的心电图改变包括：T波高尖（称为超早期T波改变），ST段抬高和（或）压低，QRS波改变，以及T波倒置"[3]。急性心肌梗死最早的改变可能是T波振幅增加、高耸和高尖。T波改变通常只持续5～30 min，随后是ST段改变，抬高和（或）压低。随着心肌梗死的进展，QRS波发生改变，包括R波振幅降低和病理性Q波形成。心肌梗死在心电图上随着时间进展将发生一系列的演变，这一连续演变被称为"动态演变"。为了描述心肌梗死不同的阶段，"早期""急性期""近期"和"陈旧期"这些传统术语已经被应用几十年。新近，按照"全球心肌梗死定义"，心肌梗死被定义为"急性"和"陈旧性"两类[4]。早期心电图改变是特征性的"超早期"T波改变和ST段抬高（见图20-1）。

followed by injury and necrosis. This event is myocardial infarction. According to "AHA/ACCF/HRS Recommendations", "The ECG changes that occur in association with acute ischemia and infarction include peaking of the T waves, referred to as hyperacute T wave changes, ST segment elevation and/or depression, changes in the QRS complex, and inverted T waves."[3] The earliest signs of acute myocardial infarction may be an increase in T wave amplitude, tall and often peaked, referred to as "hyperacute" T wave changes. These changes in T wave are usually present for only 5 to 30 minutes after the onset of infarction and are followed by ST segment changes, elevation and/or depression. As the acute myocardial infarction evolves, changes in the QRS complex include loss of R wave height and the development of pathological Q wave. Myocardial infarction may manifest in a series of changes in ECG as time goes on, referred to as the "evolution" of infarction pattern. To describe the various stages of myocardial infarction, traditional terms "early" "acute" "recent" and "old (previous or prior)" have been used for several decades. Recently, the definition of myocardial infarction includes "acute" and "prior" according to "Universal Definition of Myocardial Infarction" [4]. The manifestations of ECG in "early stage" are typically "hyperacute" T wave changes and ST segment elevation (see Fig. 20-1).

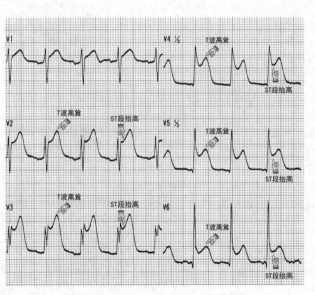

图20-1 "超早期"T波改变和ST段抬高

Fig. 20-1 "Hyperacute" T wave changes and ST segment elevation

图例21 急性前间壁心肌梗死(早期)

Case 21　Acute Anteroseptal Myocardial Infarction (Early Stage)

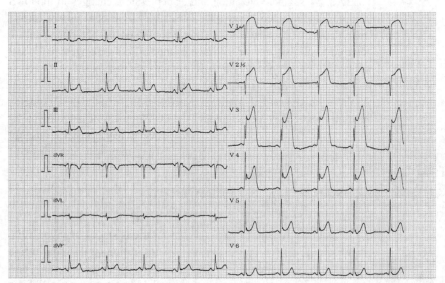

ECG Characteristics

1. HR: 65 bpm; PR: 145 ms; QRS D: 82 ms; QT/QTc: 360/375 ms; QRS axis: −11°.

2. ST segments elevation in leads V1 ~ V4 is 0.30 ~ 1.60 mV. T wave: tall and peaked in leads V1 ~ V4. There is no pathological Q wave in all leads.

ECG Interpretation

Sinus rhythm, acute anteroseptal myocardial infarction (early stage).

The most frequently used the ECG criterion for identifying acute ischemia and myocardial infarction is "ST-T criteria." According to "Third Universal Definition of Myocardial Infarction"[5], the "ST-T criteria" for the diagnosis of acute myocardial ischemia that may or may not lead to myocardial infarction includes "ST elevation" and "ST depression and T wave changes" (see Tab. 21-1). When the ST segment is elevated, the term of ST-segment-elevation myocardial infarction (STEMI) is used. The STEMI designation is contrasted with that of NSTEMI (or non-STEMI), which includes all others.

心电图特点

1. 心率: 65次/min; PR间期: 145 ms; QRS波时间: 82 ms; QT/QTc间期: 360/375 ms; QRS波电轴: −11°。

2. V1 ~ V4导联ST段抬高0.30 ~ 1.60 mV。T波在V1 ~ V4导联直立高耸。所有导联未见异常Q波。

心电图诊断与解析

诊断: 窦性心律; 急性前间壁心肌梗死

（早期）。

解析：心电图诊断心肌缺血和梗死最常用的是"ST-T标准"。根据"第三轮全球心肌梗死的定义"[5]，对于可能导致或并不导致心肌梗死的心肌缺血，"ST-T标准"包括"ST段抬高"和"ST段压低和T波改变"（见表21-1）。当有ST段抬高，称为ST段抬高心肌梗死（STEMI），与此相反，其他类型称为非ST段抬高心肌梗死。

表21-1　急性心肌缺血的心电图表现

ST抬高：相邻两个导联上新出现ST段J点抬高：除外V2和V3导联，其他所有导联抬高≥0.1 mV。V2和V3导联：男性≥40岁，≥0.2 mV；男性<40岁，≥0.25 mV；女性≥0.15 mV

ST压低和T波改变：相邻两个导联上新出现ST段水平型或下斜型压低≥0.05 mV和相邻两个导联上T波倒置≥0.1 mV伴高大R波或R/S>1

"相邻导联"是指解剖上相连的导联，即两个导联在心脏解剖位置上是相邻的。胸前导联，自右前向左侧，V1至V6导联之间依次是相邻的导联。肢体导联，自左上至右下，相邻导联依次是aVL、Ⅰ、−aVR、Ⅱ、aVF和Ⅲ导联。此心电图中ST段抬高可见于V1~V4的相邻导联，见图21-1。

Tab. 21-1　ECG Manifestations of Acute Myocardial Ischemia

ST elevation: New ST elevation at the J point in two contiguous leads with the cut point: ≥ 0.1 mV in all leads other than leads V2 ~ V3 where the following cut point apply: ≥ 0.2 mV in men ≥ 40 years; ≥ 0.25 mV in men < 40 years, or ≥ 0.15 mV in women

ST depression and T wave changes: New horizontal or down-sloping ST depression ≥ 0.05 mV in two contiguous leads/or T inversion ≥ 0.1 mV in two contiguous leads with prominent R wave or R/S ratio > 1

The "contiguous leads" indicate anatomical relationship of leads: two leads located at neighboring anatomical areas of heart. The precordial leads from V1 through V6 are "contiguous leads" from right anterior (V1) to left lateral (V6). For limb leads, from left superior-basal to right inferior, "contiguous leads" are leads from aVL, Ⅰ, −aVR, Ⅱ, aVF to Ⅲ. See Fig. 21-1 for elevated ST segments in "contiguous leads" V1 ~ V4.

图21-1　ST-T改变

Fig. 21-1　ST-T abnormalities

图例22 急性下壁心肌梗死（早期）

Case 22 Acute Inferior Myocardial Infarction (Early Stage)

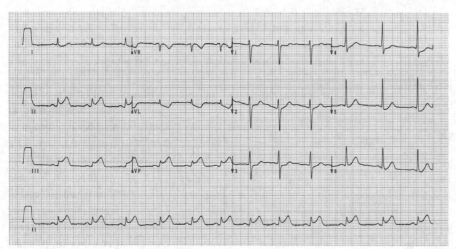

心电图特点

1. 心率：73次/min，PR间期：150 ms，QRS波时间：92 ms，QT/QTc间期：396/436 ms，QRS波电轴：54°。

2. Ⅱ、Ⅲ和aVF导联ST段抬高0.15～0.2 mV；Ⅰ和aVL导联ST段压低0.1～0.15 mV。

3. T波在Ⅱ、Ⅲ和aVF导联直立高耸，在aVL导联倒置。所有导联未见异常Q波。

心电图诊断与解析

诊断：窦性心律；急性下壁心肌梗死（早期）。

ECG Characteristics

1. HR: 73 bpm; PR: 150 ms; QRS D: 92 ms; QT/QTc: 396/436 ms; QRS axis: 54°.

2. ST segment elevation in leads Ⅱ, Ⅲ and aVF is 0.15 ~ 0.2 mV, depression in leads Ⅰ and aVL is 0.1 ~ 0.15 mV.

3. T waves are tall and peaked in leads Ⅱ, Ⅲ and aVF, and inverted in lead aVL. There is no pathological Q wave in all leads.

ECG Interpretation

Sinus rhythm, acute inferior myocardial infarction (early stage).

Locating infarction area is an important aspect of ECG evaluation of myocardial infarction. The distribution of ECG changes recorded during myocardial infarction, including ST-T abnormalities and Q wave, allows the region of infarction to be found (see Tab. 22-1). Fig. 22-1 illustrates the correlation of contiguous leads to the region involved and to the occluded vessel. In this ECG, tall and peaked T wave and elevated ST segment in leads Ⅱ, Ⅲ and aVF have been seen and pathological Q wave have not been seen in all leads, indicating early stage of acute inferior myocardial infarction (see Fig. 22-2).

解析：心肌梗死定位是心电图评判心肌梗死的重要部分。心肌梗死中ST-T改变和Q波等心电图变化的分布可用于定位梗死部位，见表22-1。图22-1示相邻导联与梗死部位和血管闭塞之间的相关性。此心电图中Ⅱ、Ⅲ和aVF可见T波高耸和ST段抬高，所有导联未见异常Q波。因此诊断为急性下壁心肌梗死（早期），见图22-2。

表22-1　心肌梗死的定位诊断/Location of Myocardial Infarction

部位/Site	导联/Leads
前间壁/Anteroseptal	V1～V3 或 V1～V4
前壁/Anterior	V3 和 V4 或 V3～V5
侧壁/Lateral	Ⅰ、aVL、V5 和 V6
广泛前壁/Extensive anterior	V1～V6 或 Ⅰ、aVL 和 V1～V6
下壁/Inferior	Ⅱ、Ⅲ 和 aVF
后壁/Posterior	V7～V9
右心室/Right ventricular	V1～V5R

注：V5R是右胸对应V5的部位(Note: V5R is corresponding points of V5 on the right side)

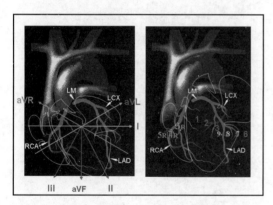

图22-1　相邻导联与梗死部位和相关冠脉

Fig. 22-1　Correlation of contiguous leads to the occluded vessel involved

注：LM：左主干；LAD：左前降支；LCX：左回旋支；RCA：右冠脉

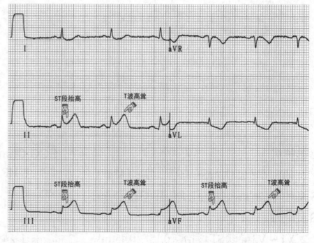

图22-2　ST-T改变

Fig. 22-2　ST-T abnormalities

图例23　急性前间壁心肌梗死

Case 23　Acute Anteroseptal Myocardial Infarction

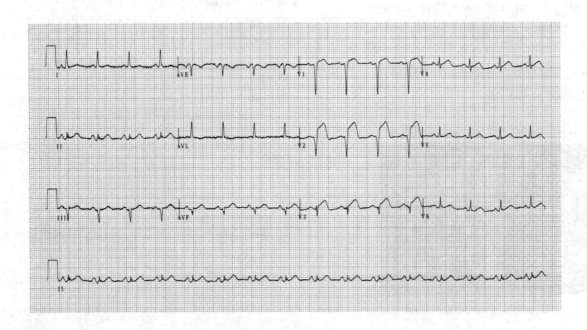

心电图特点

1. 心 率：95次/min；PR间 期：142 ms；QRS波时间：76 ms；QT/QTc间期：332/417 ms；QRS波电轴：−11°。

2. V1 ~ V3导联ST段抬高0.15 ~ 0.45 mV。T波在V1 ~ V3导联直立高耸，在Ⅰ和aVL导联低平。QRS波V1和V2导联呈QS型，V3

ECG Characteristics

1. HR: 95 bpm; PR: 142 ms; QRS D: 76 ms; QT/QTc: 332/417 ms; QRS axis: −11°.

2. ST segments elevation in leads V1 ~ V3 is 0.15 ~ 0.45 mV. T waves are tall and peaked in leads V1 ~ V3, and low and flat in leads Ⅰ and aVL. QRS complexes are QS pattern in leads V1 and V2, and rS pattern in lead V3.

导联呈 rS 型。

心电图诊断与解析

诊断：窦性心律；急性前间壁心肌梗死。

解析：随着急性心肌梗死的进展，记录电极周围的心肌活力降低或坏死，在心电图上 QRS 波将发生改变，包括 R 波振幅降低和病理性 Q 波形成。正常 QRS 波代表不同部位心肌除极的综合电势。在心肌梗死中，坏死部位心肌无电活动，综合除极电势背离该部位，在心电图上形成 Q 波。按照传统的分期诊断，属于"急性期"心肌梗死。此心电图中，V1 和 V2 导联 QRS 波呈 QS 型，即 R 波消失和 Q 波形成。心电图诊断为急性前间壁心肌梗死。QRS 波形态识别见图 23-1。

ECG Interpretation

Sinus rhythm, acute anteroseptal myocardial infarction.

As a result of the loss of viable myocardium or necrosis beneath the recording electrode when acute myocardial infarction evolves, QRS complex changes, including loss of R wave height and the development of pathological Q wave. The normal QRS complex represents the resultant of the electrical forces generated from the various portions of the myocardium during ventricular depolarization. In myocardial infarction, the area of necrosis becomes electrically silent. The balance of the ventricular depolarization forces tends to point away from this area and Q wave develops on the ECG. According to traditional terms, this stage is the "acute" stage of myocardial infarction. In this ECG, QRS complexes lose R waves and develop Q waves, resulting in QS pattern in leads V1 and V2. The ECG interpretation is acute anteroseptal myocardial infarction. For the patterns of QRS complex, see Fig. 23-1.

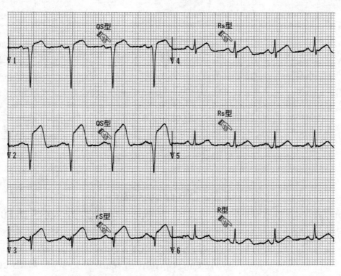

图 23-1　QRS 波形态

Fig. 23-1　Patterns of QRS complex

图例24　急性前壁心肌梗死

Case 24　Acute Anterior Myocardial Infarction

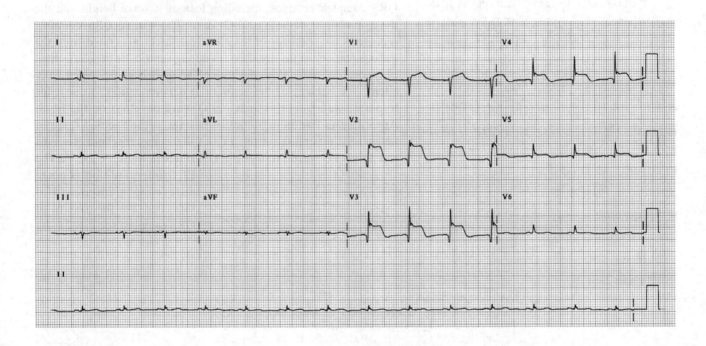

心电图特点

1. 心　率: 86次/min; PR间　期: 120 ms;
QRS波时间: 80 ms; QT/QTc间期: 304/363 ms;
QRS波电轴: 5°。

2. V1 ~ V5导联ST段抬高0.10 ~ 0.55 mV。
T波在V1 ~ V5导联直立。QRS波V1导联呈

ECG Characteristics

1. HR: 86 bpm; PR: 120 ms; QRS D: 80 ms; QT/QTc: 304/363 ms;
QRS axis: 5°.

2. ST segments elevation in leads V1 ~ V5 is 0.10 ~ 0.55 mV. T
waves are upright in leads V1 ~ V5. QRS complexes are rS pattern in
lead V1 and qR pattern in leads V2 ~ V5; Q wave amplitude is $\geq 25\,\%$
of R wave amplitude; the amplitude of QRS complex is < 0.5 mV in

rS 型，V2 ~ V5 导联呈 qR 型，Q 波 ≥ R 波振幅的 25%；肢体导联 QRS 波振幅 <0.5 mV。

心电图诊断与解析

诊断：窦性心律；急性前壁心肌梗死；肢体导联低电压。

解析：作为心肌坏死的征象，Q 波通常出现在急性心肌梗死症状发生后 1 ~ 2 h 内。病理性 Q 波的定义是，时间 ≥ 40 ms 或振幅 ≥ 同导联 R 波振幅的 25%（1/4）。此心电图中，V2 ~ V4 导联 Q 波 ≥ R 波振幅的 25%（见图 24-1），ST 段仍抬高，T 波仍直立，因此心电图诊断为急性前壁心肌梗死。另外肢体导联低电压的定义是 QRS 波（R+S）振幅 <0.5 mV。

limb leads.

ECG Interpretation

Sinus rhythm, acute Anterior myocardial infarction, low voltage in limb leads.

In general, as a marker of myocardial necrosis, Q wave may develop within one to two hours of the onset of the symptoms of acute myocardial infarction. Pathologic Q wave is usually defined as duration ≥ 40 ms or ≥ 25 % (1/4) of R wave amplitude in the same lead. In this ECG, Q waves are ≥ 25 % of R waves in leads V2 ~ V4 (see Fig. 24-1). ST segments are still elevated and T waves are upright in leads V1 ~ V5. The ECG interpretation is acute anterior myocardial infarction. Additionally, low voltage in limb leads is defined as the sum of R and S wave amplitude is < 0.5 mV for the QRS complex.

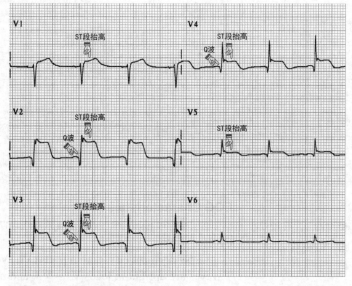

图 24-1　病理性 Q 波和 ST-T 改变

Fig. 24-1　Pathologic Q wave and ST-T abnormalities

图例25　急性前侧壁心肌梗死

Case 25　Acute Anterolateral Myocardial Infarction

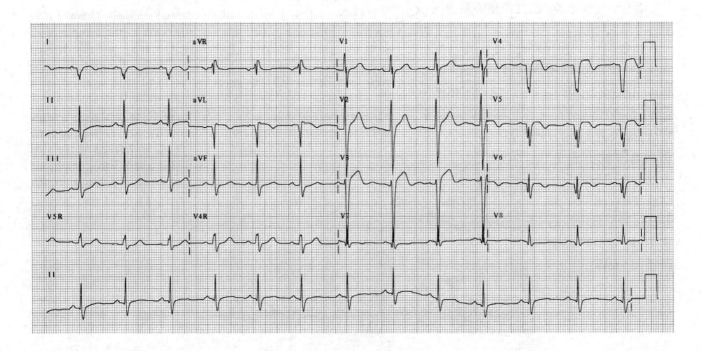

心电图特点

1. 心率：79次/min；PR间期：166 ms；QRS波时间：107 ms；QT/QTc间期：397/455 ms；QRS波电轴：158°。

2. aVL、V3 ~ V5导联ST段抬高0.10 ~ 0.25 mV。T波在V1 ~ V3导联直立，在V4 ~

ECG Characteristics

1. HR: 79 bpm; PR: 166 ms; QRS D: 107 ms; QT/QTc: 397/455 ms; QRS axis: 158°.

2. ST segment elevation in leads aVL, V3 ~ V5 is 0.10 ~ 0.25 mV. T waves are upright in leads V1 ~ V3, and inverted in leads V4 ~ V6. QRS complexes are QS pattern in leads Ⅰ, aVL, V4 and V5; R wave in lead V3 < R wave in lead V2; qrS pattern in lead V6; qRs pattern

V6导联倒置。QRS波在Ⅰ、aVL、V4和V5导联呈QS型，V3导联R波＜V2导联R波，V6导联呈qrS型。V7和V8导联呈qRs型。

心电图诊断与解析

诊断：窦性心律；急性前侧壁心肌梗死；电轴右偏。

解析：正常时，胸前导联中QRS波由主波向下转为主波向上。V1或V2导联由小r波开始，至V5或V6导联，逐渐增大至大R波。V1或V2导联至V5或V6导联R波不逐渐增大，提示胸前导联R波递增不良。心肌梗死时，R波振幅降低可以引起胸前导联R波递增不良。此心电图中，V3导联R波小于V2导联R波（见图25-1），这一异常征象提示V3导联R波振幅降低。结合其他异常征象，包括Ⅰ、aVL、V4和V5导联呈QS型，V6导联呈qrS型和ST段抬高，心电图诊断为急性前侧壁心肌梗死。

in lead V7 and V8.

ECG Interpretation

Sinus rhythm, acute anterolateral myocardial infarction, right axis deviation.

Normally, QRS complex changes from mainly negative to mainly positive in the precordial leads. Small r wave begins in lead V1 or V2 and progress in size to R wave in lead V5 or V6. Abnormal precordial R wave progression is indicated when the R wave dose not progress in size from lead V1 or V2 to V5 or V6. In myocardial infarction, loss of R wave height may cause abnormal precordial R wave progression. In this ECG, R wave in lead V3 is smaller than that in lead V2 (see Fig. 25–1). That abnormal sign indicates that loss of R wave height in lead V3. Combining other abnormal signs, including QS pattern in leads Ⅰ, aVL, V4 and V5 and qrS pattern in lead V6, and ST segments elevate, the ECG interpretation is acute anterolateral myocardial infarction.

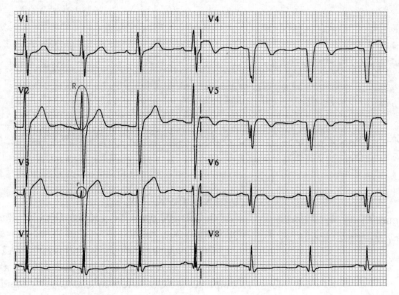

图 25-1　R波振幅改变

Fig. 25-1　Changes of R wave amplitude

图例26 急性广泛前壁心肌梗死

Case 26 Acute Extensive Anterior Myocardial Infarction

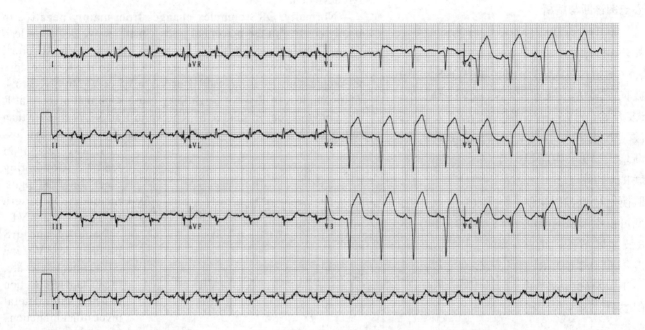

心电图特点

1. 心 率: 100次/min; PR间 期: 136 ms; QRS波时间: 78 ms; QT/QTc间期: 350/451 ms; QRS波电轴: -41°。

2. Ⅰ、aVL、V1 ~ V6导联ST段抬高 0.10 ~ 0.60 mV。T波在Ⅰ、aVL、V1 ~ V6导联直立。QRS波在V1 ~ V5导联呈QS型,V6

ECG Characteristics

1. HR: 100 bpm; PR: 136 ms; QRS D: 78 ms; QT/QTc: 350/451 ms; QRS axis: -41°.

2. ST segments elevation in leads Ⅰ, aVL and V1 ~ V6 is 0.10 ~ 0.60 mV. T waves are upright in leads Ⅰ, aVL and V1 ~ V6. QRS complexes are QS pattern in leads V1 ~ V5 and qrS pattern in lead V6.

ECG Interpretation

Sinus rhythm, acute extensive anterior myocardial infarction,

导联呈 qrS 型。

心电图诊断与解析

诊断：窦性心律；急性广泛前壁心肌梗死；电轴左偏。

解析：心脏前壁部位是心肌梗死最常见部位，心电图诊断前壁部位心肌梗死，可进一步分为前间壁、前壁和侧壁。当 Ⅰ 和 aVL 导联、V1～V4 导联，有时至 V6 导联出现 ST 段抬高，则提示广泛前壁心肌梗死。前壁部位的心肌梗死，提示冠脉左前降支病变。左前降支近端闭塞可以造成广泛的心电图异常，即广泛前壁心肌梗死。此心电图中，Ⅰ、aVL、V1～V6 导联出现 ST 段抬高，V1～V5 导联出现病理性 Q 波（见图 26-1），因此心电图诊断为急性广泛前壁心肌梗死。

left axis deviation.

The anterior aspect of heart is the area most commonly subject to infarction. The ECG diagnosis of myocardial infarction location at the anterior aspect may be further differentiated into anteroseptal, anterior and lateral wall infarction. The presences of ST segment elevation in leads Ⅰ and aVL, as well as in leads V1～V4 and sometimes in V6, suggest an extensive anterior wall infarction. The anterior aspect infarction is the indicator of left anterior descending artery disease. Proximal left anterior descending coronary artery occlusion tends to produce the most widespread ECG abnormalities, i.e., extensive anterior myocardial infarction. In this ECG, ST segment elevation is present in leads Ⅰ, aVL and V1～V6, and pathologic Q wave is present in leads V1～V5 (see Fig. 26-1), thus ECG interpretation is acute extensive anterior myocardial infarction.

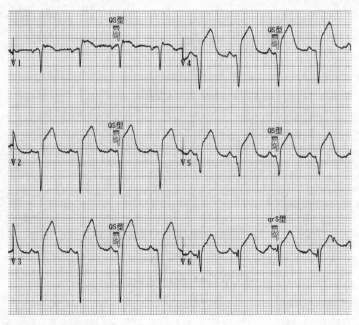

图 26-1 病理性 Q 波

Fig. 26-1 Pathologic Q wave

图例27　急性下壁心肌梗死

Case 27　Acute Inferior Myocardial Infarction

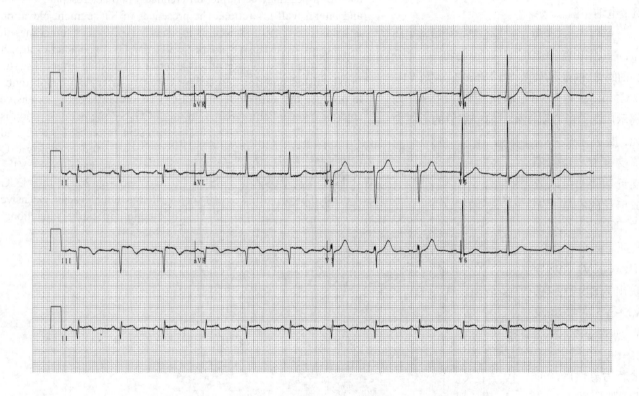

心电图特点

1. 心率: 74次/min; PR间期: 160 ms; QRS波时间: 82 ms; QT/QTc间期: 410/455 ms; QRS波电轴: −27°。

ECG Characteristics

1. HR: 74 bpm; PR: 160 ms; QRS D: 82 ms; QT/QTc: 410/455 ms; QRS axis: −27°.

2. ST segments elevation in leads Ⅱ, Ⅲ and aVF is 0.10 ~ 0.15 mV. T waves are inverted in leads Ⅱ, Ⅲ and aVF. QRS complexes are Qr

2. Ⅱ、Ⅲ和aVF导联ST段抬高0.10～0.15 mV。T波在Ⅱ、Ⅲ和aVF导联倒置。QRS波在Ⅱ导联呈Qr型，在Ⅲ和aVF导联呈QS型。

心电图诊断与解析

诊断：窦性心律；急性下壁心肌梗死。

解析：心脏的下壁部位也是心肌梗死常见部位，如前所述（图例21和22），下壁解剖上相邻导联依次是Ⅱ、aVF和Ⅲ导联。此心电图中，Ⅱ、aVF和Ⅲ导联出现ST段抬高和病理性Q波（见图27-1），心电图诊断为急性下壁心肌梗死。随着心肌梗死的进展，抬高的ST段回落，T波开始倒置。T波倒置可以持续存在数月，偶尔可持续存在而成为永久的梗死征象。下壁心肌梗死通常与右冠状动脉和左回旋支病变有关。

pattern in lead Ⅱ and QS pattern in leads Ⅲ and aVF.

ECG Interpretation

Sinus rhythm, acute inferior myocardial infarction.

The inferior aspect of heart is also commonly subject to infarction. As mentioned before (case 21 and 22), inferior "contiguous leads" are leads from Ⅱ, aVF to Ⅲ. In this ECG, ST segment elevation and pathologic Q are present in leads Ⅱ, aVF and Ⅲ (see Fig. 27-1). The ECG interpretation is acute inferior myocardial infarction. As myocardial infarction evolves, ST segment elevation diminishes and T wave begins to invert. T wave inversion may persist for many months and occasionally remain as a permanent sign of infarction. Inferior myocardial infarction is usually associated with disease in the right coronary or distal circumflex artery.

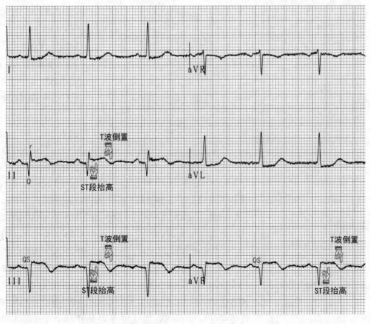

图27-1 病理性Q波和T波倒置

Fig. 27-1 Pathologic Q wave and inverted T wave

图例28　急性后壁心肌梗死

Case 28　Acute Posterior Myocardial Infarction

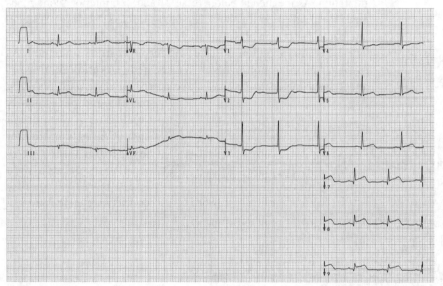

ECG Characteristics

1. HR: 62 bpm; PR: 178 ms; QRS D: 92 ms; QT/QTc: 410/415 ms; QRS axis: 28°.

2. ST segments depression in leads V1~V3 is 0.20 ~ 0.30 mV, and elevation in leads V7 ~ V9 is 0.10 ~ 0.15 mV. T waves are upright in leads V1 ~ V9. QRS complexes are Rs pattern in leads V1 ~ V3 and qR pattern in leads V7 ~ V9.

ECG Interpretation

Sinus rhythm, acute posterior myocardial infarction.

The ECG changes in myocardial infarction can be divided into indicative changes and reciprocal changes (see Fig. 28–1). ST segment elevation, loss of R wave height and development of pathological Q wave are indicative changes on the side directly over the infarction area. ST segment depression, upright T wave and increase of R wave height may be reciprocal changes on the side opposite to the infarction area. In this ECG, dominant R wave in leads V1 ~ V3 with ST segment depression and upright T wave suggest acute posterior myocardial infarction. Provided with additional leads V7 ~ V9, where ST segment elevation and Q wave are seen (see Fig. 28–2), the diagnosis is confirmed. Not all of posterior myocardial infarction has such changes in 12-lead ECG. The standard 12-lead ECG does not include posterior leads

心电图特点

1. 心率：62次/min；PR间期：178 ms；QRS波时间：92 ms；QT/QTc间期：410/416 ms；QRS波电轴：28°。

2. V1 ~ V3导联ST段压低0.20 ~ 0.30 mV，V7 ~ V9导联ST段抬高0.10 ~ 0.15 mV。T波在V1 ~ V9导联直立。QRS波在V1 ~ V3导联呈Rs型，在V7 ~ V9导联呈qR型。

心电图诊断与解析

诊断：窦性心律；急性后壁心肌梗死。

解析：急性心肌梗死的心电图改变可以分为直接改变和对应改变（见图28-1）。ST段抬高、R波振幅降低和病理性Q波形成是面对梗死部位的直接改变。ST段压低、T波直立和R波振幅增高，可以是背对梗死部位的对应改变。此心电图中，V1～V3导联高大R波，伴有ST段压低和T波直立，提示急性后壁心肌梗死。附加V7～V9导联可见ST段抬高和Q波，诊断确立（见图28-2）。并非所有的后壁心肌梗死在12导联心电图中有如此改变。标准12导联心电图并不直接检测左心室后基底部和侧壁部位，不附加后壁导联（V7～V9）常可能遗漏诊断。因此在心肌梗死或其他急性冠脉综合征，或有缺血性胸痛和初次心电图记录不能明确诊断时，推荐附加后壁导联。

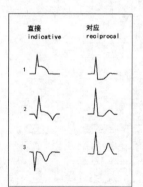

图28-1 直接和对应改变

Fig. 28-1 Indicative changes and reciprocal changes

(V7 ~ V9) and thus cannot directly examine the posterior basal and lateral aspect of the left ventricle, leading to non-diagnostic ECG for posterior myocardial infarction. Therefore the use of additional posterior leads can be recommended during infarction or other acute coronary syndrome and for patients with ischemic chest pain and a non-diagnostic initial ECG.

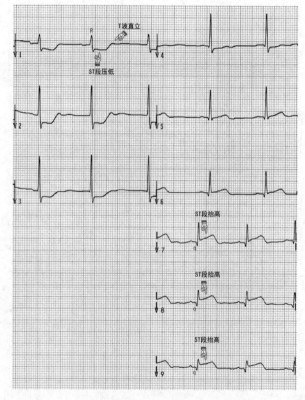

图28-2 后壁心肌梗死的心电图改变

Fig. 28-2 ECG changes in posterior myocardial infarction

图例29　急性下壁和后侧壁心肌梗死

Case 29　Acute Inferior and Posterolateral Myocardial Infarction

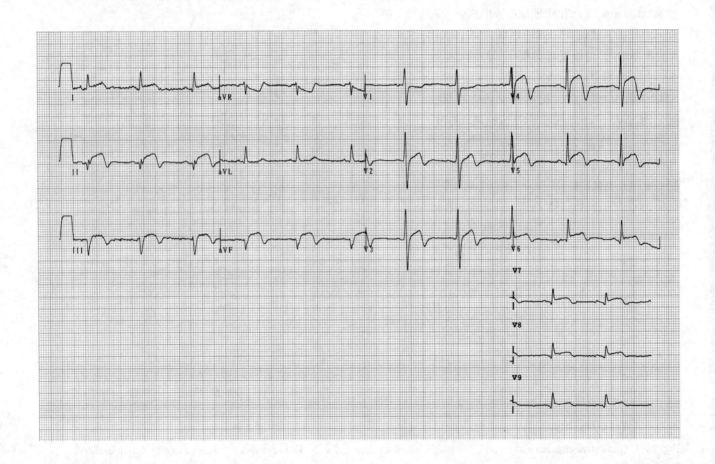

心电图特点

1. 心率：66次/min；PR间期：138 ms；QRS波时间：102 ms；QT/QTc间期：434/454 ms；QRS波电轴：−31°。

2. Ⅰ、Ⅱ、Ⅲ、aVF和V4～V9导联ST段抬高0.10～0.20 mV，aVR和V1导联ST段压低0.10 mV。T波在Ⅰ、aVL和V1导联直立，在Ⅱ、Ⅲ、aVF和V2～V9导联倒置。QRS波在Ⅱ导联呈qrs型，Q波>R波。

心电图诊断与解析

诊断：窦性心律；急性下壁和后侧壁心肌梗死；电轴左偏。

解析：急性后壁心肌梗死常合并见于心脏下壁部位，因此对于下壁心肌梗死强烈推荐附加记录后壁导联。附加后壁导联位于第五肋间水平，V7导联在左腋后线，V8导联在肩胛骨中线，V9导联在左脊柱旁。ST段抬高的阈值推荐为0.05 mV[3]。此心电图中，Ⅱ、Ⅲ和aVF导联ST段抬高，同时V4～V6导联ST段抬高，V1导联ST段压低和T波直立，所有征象提示梗死累及后壁。附加V7～V9导联，可见ST段抬高和Q波，诊断确立（见图29-1）。下壁合并后侧壁心肌梗死，强烈提示左回旋支病变。

ECG Characteristics

1. HR: 66 bpm; PR: 138 ms; QRS D: 102 ms; QT/QTc: 434/454 ms; QRS axis: −31°.

2. ST segments elevation in leads Ⅰ, Ⅱ, Ⅲ, aVF and V4 ~ V9 is 0.10 ~ 0.20 mV, and depression in leads aVR and V1 is 0.10 mV.T waves are upright in leads Ⅰ, aVL and V1, and inverted in leads Ⅱ, Ⅲ, aVF and V2 ~ V9. QRS complex is qrs pattern in lead Ⅱ; Q wave is > R wave.

ECG Interpretation

Sinus rhythm, acute inferior and posterolateral myocardial infarction, left axis deviation.

Acute posterior myocardial infarctions are often seen with inferior aspect of heart. Therefore the use of additional posterior leads is strongly recommended in patients with inferior infarction. The additional posterior leads are at the fifth intercostal space, V7 at the left posterior axillary line, V8 at the left mid-scapular line, and V9 at the left paraspinal border. The threshold value of ST segment elevation in leads V7 ~ V9 is recommended to be 0.05 mV.[3] In this ECG, ST segment elevation in leads Ⅱ, Ⅲ and aVF, as well as leads V4 ~ V6 and ST segment depression in lead V1 with upright T wave, all evidences suggest posterior wall may be involved. Provided with additional leads V7~V9, where ST segment elevation and Q wave are seen (see Fig. 29-1), the diagnosis is confirmed. Inferior combined with posterolateral myocardial infarction highly suggests disease in circumflex artery.

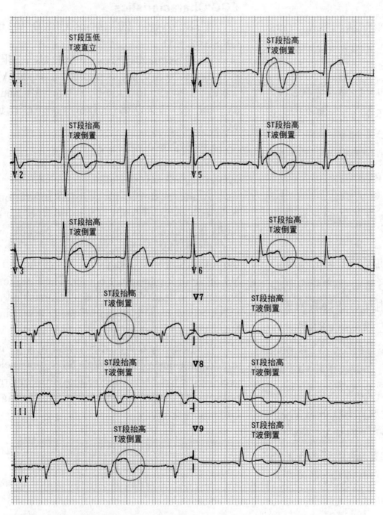

图 29-1 后壁心肌梗死的心电图改变

Fig. 29-1 ECG changes in posterior myocardial infarction

图例30 急性前间壁、下壁和右心室心肌梗死

Case 30 Acute Anteroseptal, Inferior and Right Ventricular Myocardial Infarction

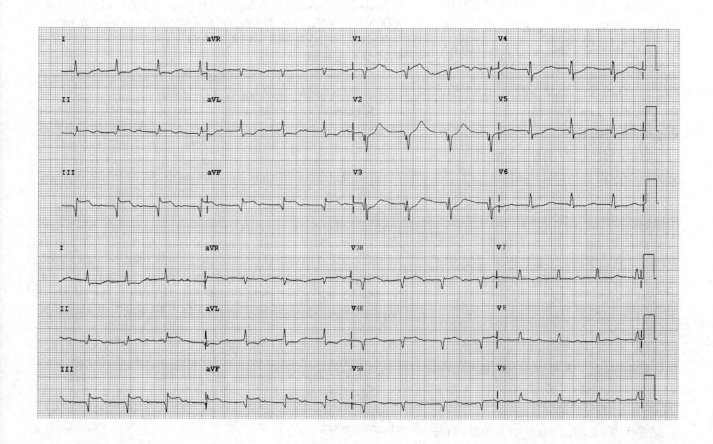

心电图特点

1. 心率：85次/min；PR间期：304 ms；QRS波时间：100 ms；QT/QTc间期：372/442 ms；QRS波电轴：29°。

2. Ⅱ、Ⅲ和aVF导联ST段抬高0.10 ~ 0.20 mV，V3R ~ V5R导联ST段抬高0.05 ~ 0.10 mV，Ⅰ和aVL导联ST段压低0.10 mV。T波在Ⅱ、Ⅲ、aVF、V3R ~ V5R和V1 ~ V3导联直立。QRS波在Ⅱ、Ⅲ、aVF、V3R ~ V5R和V1 ~ V3导联呈Qr或QS型。

心电图诊断与解析

诊断：窦性心律；急性前间壁、下壁和右心室心肌梗死；一度房室传导阻滞。

解析：右心室心肌梗死常伴发于下壁心肌梗死，也可伴发于部分前壁心肌梗死，单独右心室发生梗死极少。由于标准12导联心电图不是右心室病变的敏感指标，右心室梗死可能被漏诊。在12导联心电图中，下壁心肌梗死提示右心室梗死的征象是V1导联ST段抬高。因此下壁心肌梗死可疑右心室梗死时，应记录右胸导联V3R和V4R。右胸导联包括V3R、V4R、V5R和V6R，相对应V3、V4、V5和V6导联部位点，但位于右胸壁。V3R和V4R导联ST段抬高的阈值是0.05 mV[3]。此心电图中，Ⅱ、Ⅲ和aVF导联ST段抬高，V1导联ST段抬高和T波直立，所有征象提示梗死

ECG Characteristics

1. HR: 85 bpm; PR: 304 ms; QRS D: 100 ms; QT/QTc: 372/442 ms; QRS axis: 29°.

2. ST segments elevation in leads Ⅱ, Ⅲ and aVF is 0.10 ~ 0.20 mV, elevation in V3R ~ V5R is 0.05 ~ 0.10 mV, and depression in leads Ⅰ and aVL is 0.10 mV. T waves are upright in leads Ⅱ, Ⅲ, aVF, V3R ~ V5R, and V1 ~ V3. QRS complexes are Qr or QS pattern in leads Ⅱ, Ⅲ, aVF, V3R ~ V5R, and V1 ~ V3.

ECG Interpretation

Sinus rhythm, acute anteroseptal, inferior and right ventricular myocardial infarction, first degree A–V block.

Right ventricular infarction is often associated with inferior infarction. It may also complicate with anterior infarction but rarely occurs as an isolated infarction. Right ventricular infarction may be missed as standard 12-lead ECG is not a sensitive indicator of right ventricular damage. In the standard 12-lead ECG, right ventricular infarction is indicated by signs of inferior infarction associated with ST segment elevation in lead V1. Therefore in patient with inferior and suspected right ventricular infarction, right precordial leads V3R and V4R should be recorded. These right precordial leads include V3R, V4R, V5R and V6R, which use the corresponding points to the V3, V4, V5 and V6 but on the right side of the chest wall. The threshold for abnormal ST segment elevation in V3R and V4R should be 0.05 mV.[3] In this ECG, ST segment elevation in leads Ⅱ, Ⅲ and aVF and elevation in lead V1 with upright T wave, all evidences suggest right ventricular may be involved. Provided with additional leads V3R ~ V5R, where ST segment elevation and Q wave are seen (see Fig. 30–1), the diagnosis is confirmed. Inferior combined with right ventricular myocardial infarction strongly suggests disease in right coronary artery.

累及右心室。附加V3R ~ V5R导联,可见ST段抬高和Q波,诊断确立(见图30-1)。下壁合并右心室心肌梗死,强烈提示右冠脉病变。

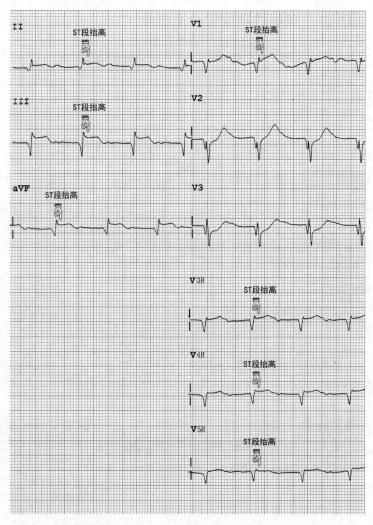

图 30-1 ST段抬高

Fig. 30-1 ST segment elevation

图例31　陈旧性前间壁心肌梗死

Case 31　Old Anteroseptal Myocardial Infarction

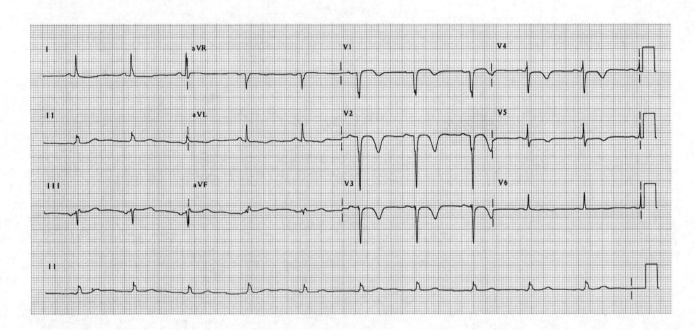

心电图特点

1.　心　率：63次/min；PR间　期：166 ms；QRS波时间：94 ms；QT/QTc间期：428/438 ms；QRS波电轴：23°。

2.　QRS波在V1和V2导联呈QS型，在V3和V4导联呈rS型。所有导联ST段无抬高。T波在V1～V5导联倒置，在Ⅰ、aVL和

ECG Characteristics

1. HR: 63 bpm; PR: 166 ms; QRS D: 94 ms; QT/QTc: 428/438 ms; QRS axis: 23°.

2. QRS complexes are QS pattern in leads V1 and V2, and rS pattern in leads V3 and V4. ST segments close to the isoelectric line in all leads. T waves are inverted in leads V1 ~ V5 and low in leads Ⅰ, aVL and V6.

V6导联低平。

心电图诊断与解析

诊断：窦性心律；陈旧性前间壁心肌梗死。

解析：当梗死完全形成后，Q波达到最深。当ST段开始向等电位线回复，出现对称倒置的T波。随着ST段回落，T波倒置逐渐加深，然后倒置的T波开始回复。当ST段回到等电位线和T波回复，进入这阶段称为"陈旧期"，代表心肌梗死痊愈。Q波成为心肌坏死的永久性征象，偶尔T波倒置也成为心肌梗死永久征象。此心电图中，V1和V2导联呈QS型，ST段位于等电位线，T波倒置（见图31-1），提示陈旧性前间壁心肌梗死。

ECG Interpretation

Sinus rhythm, old anteroseptal myocardial infarction.

When the infarction has fully evolved, the Q wave reaches maximal depth. As the ST segment begins to return to the isoelectric line, symmetrical inversion of the T wave appears. The inverted T wave becomes progressively deeper as ST segment deviation subsides. Then the inverted T wave begins to revert. When the ST segment has returned to the isoelectric line and the inverted T wave has reverted, the condition enters the "old" stage, meaning the myocardial infarction is healed. Q wave acts as a permanent marker of necrosis and T wave inversion occasionally remains as a permanent sign of infarction. In this ECG, QS pattern in leads V1 and V2, ST segment at the isoelectric line and T wave inverted (see Fig. 31-1) suggest old or prior anteroseptal myocardial infarction.

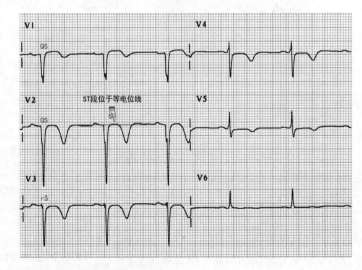

图31-1 ST段位于等电位线

Fig. 31-1 ST segment at the isoelectric line

图例32　陈旧性前壁心肌梗死

Case 32　Old Anterior Myocardial Infarction

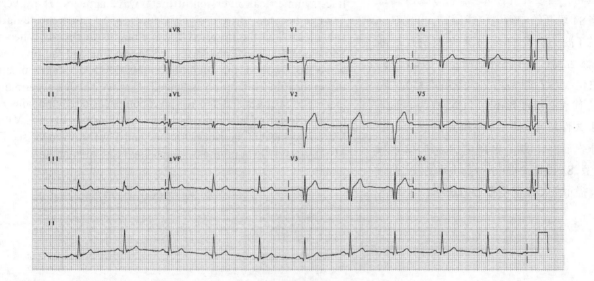

心电图特点

1. 心率: 64次/min; PR间期: 152 ms; QRS波时间: 101 ms; QT/QTc间期: 373/385 ms; QRS波电轴: 73°。

2. QRS波在V1导联呈rS型, 在V2导联呈QS型, 在V5和V6导联呈qR型; V3和V4导联Q波≥R波振幅的25%。所有导联无ST段抬高。T波在V1 ~ V3导联直立。

ECG Characteristics

1. HR: 64 bpm; PR: 152 ms; QRS D: 101 ms; QT/QTc: 373/385 ms; QRS axis: 73°.

2. QRS complexes are rS pattern in lead V1, QS pattern in lead V2, and qR pattern in leads V5 and V6; Q wave is ≥ 25% of R wave amplitude in leads V3 and V4. ST segments close to the isoelectric line in all leads. T waves are upright in leads V1 ~ V3.

ECG Interpretation

Sinus rhythm, old anterior myocardial infarction.

Normally, QRS complex changes from mainly negative to

心电图诊断与解析

诊断：窦性心律；陈旧性前壁心肌梗死。

解析：正常时，胸前导联中QRS波由主波向下转为主波向上。此心电图中，V1导联有R波而V2导联无R波，V3和V4导联Q波≥R波振幅的25%（见图32-1），提示前壁心肌梗死。在一些导联中，Q波或QS型是确诊陈旧性心肌梗死的征象[5]（见表32-1）。当Q波出现在多个或一组导联中，心电图诊断心肌梗死的特异性达到最高。

表32-1　与陈旧性心肌梗死有关的心电图改变

V2 ~ V3导联中任何导联有≥0.02 s的Q波或V2和V3呈QS型
Ⅰ、Ⅱ、aVL、aVF或V4 ~ V6导联中，任何两个相邻导联（Ⅰ、aVL；V4 ~ V6；Ⅱ、Ⅲ、aVF），Q波≥0.03 s和深度≥0.1 mV或QS型*
无传导异常，V1和V2导联R波≥0.04 s和R/S≥1，伴有一致的直立T波

注：V7 ~ V9导联的诊断标准相同。

mainly positive in precordial leads. In this ECG, the presence of R wave in lead V1 and the absence of it in lead V2 (see Fig. 32-1), Q waves are ≥ 25% of R waves amplitude in leads V3 and V4, indicate anterior myocardial infarction. Q wave or QS pattern in some leads is pathognomonic of a prior myocardial infarction[5] (see Tab. 32-1). The specificity of the ECG diagnosis for myocardial infarction is greatest when Q waves occur in several leads or lead groupings.

Tab. 32-1　ECG Changes Associated with Prior Myocardial

Any Q wave in leads V2 ~ V3 ≥ 0.02 s or QS complex in leads V2 and V3
Q wave ≥ 0.03 s and ≥ 0.1 mV deep or QS complex in leads Ⅰ, Ⅱ, aVL, aVF or V4 ~ V6 in any two leads of a contiguous lead grouping (Ⅰ, aVL; V4 ~ V6; Ⅱ, Ⅲ, aVF)*
R wave ≥ 0.04 s in V1 ~ V2 and R/S ≥ 1 with a concordant positive T wave in absence of conduction defect

Note: The same criteria are used for supplemental leads V7 ~ V9.

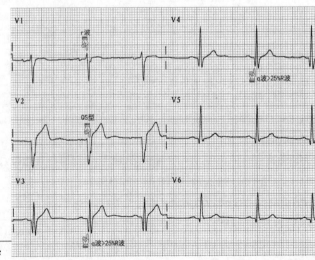

图32-1　病理性Q波

Fig. 32-1　Pathologic Q wave

图例 33 陈旧性广泛前壁心肌梗死

Case 33 Old Extensive Anterior Myocardial Infarction

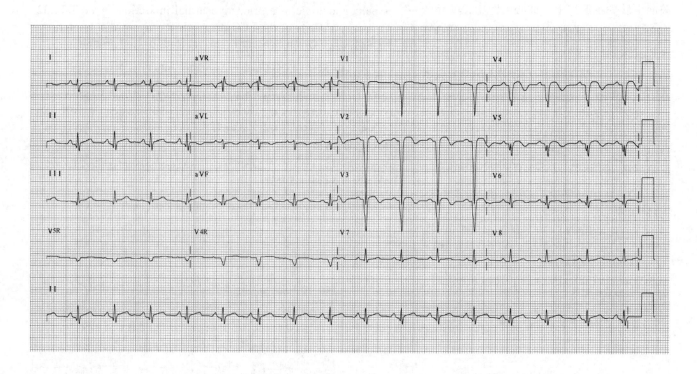

心电图特点

1. 心 率: 97次/min; PR间 期: 152 ms;
QRS波时间: 83 ms; QT/QTc间期: 337/428 ms;
QRS波电轴: 118°。

2. QRS波 在 V1 ~ V5导 联 呈 QS型, V6

ECG Characteristics

1. HR: 97 bpm; PR: 152 ms; QRS D: 83 ms; QT/QTc: 337/428 ms;
QRS axis: 118°.

2. QRS complexes are QS pattern in leads V1 ~ V5 and qRs
pattern in lead V6. ST segments close to the isoelectric line in leads
V1 ~ V6. T waves are inverted in leads V1 ~ V5.

导联呈 qRs 型。V1 ~ V6 导联 ST 段接近等电位线。T 波在 V1 ~ V5 导联倒置。

心电图诊断与解析

诊断：窦性心律；陈旧性广泛前壁心肌梗死；电轴右偏。

解析：病理性或异常 Q 波，无 ST 段抬高，提示陈旧性心肌梗死。此心电图中，V1 ~ V5 导联存在病理性 Q 波，ST 段接近等电位线，应该考虑陈旧性心肌梗死（见图 33-1）。心电图诊断梗死时期，也可根据出现梗死症状的时间来判断。当梗死广泛时，Q 波是坏死的永久性征象。另外，左心室大面积梗死是本心电图出现电轴右偏的原因。

ECG Interpretation

Sinus rhythm, old extensive anterior myocardial infarction, right axis deviation.

Presence of pathological or abnormal Q wave in leads without ST segment elevation is suggestive of old myocardial infarction. In this ECG, pathological Q waves present and ST segments close to isoelectric line in leads V1 ~ V5 (see Fig. 33-1); thus, old myocardial infarction should be considered. Interpretation of the infarction stage in ECG may also be determined according to the time since the onset of infarction symptoms. When myocardial infarction is extensive, Q wave acts as a permanent marker of necrosis. In addition, the large infarction area in the left ventricular is the cause of right axis deviation in this ECG.

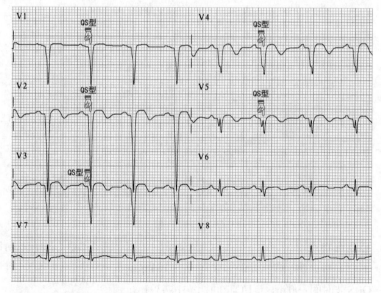

图 33-1　病理性 Q 波

Fig. 33-1　Pathologic Q wave

图例34　陈旧性下壁心肌梗死

Case 34　Old Inferior Myocardial Infarction

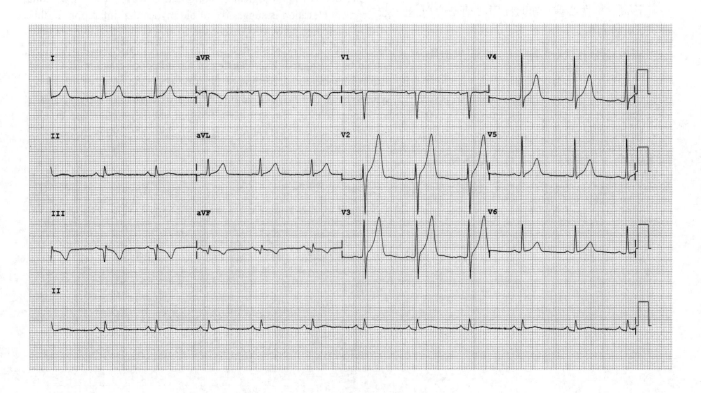

心电图特点

1. 心　率: 67次/min; PR间　期: 164 ms;
QRS波时间: 90 ms; QT/QTc间期: 416/439 ms;
QRS波电轴: 5°。

ECG Characteristics

1. HR: 67 bpm; PR: 164 ms; QRS D: 90 ms; QT/QTc: 416/439 ms; QRS axis: 5°.

2. QRS complexes are qR or Qr pattern in leads Ⅱ, Ⅲ and aVF, Q wave is ≥ 25 % of R wave amplitude in leads Ⅲ and aVF.

2. QRS波在Ⅱ、Ⅲ和aVF导联呈qR或Qr型；Ⅲ和aVF导联Q波大于R波25%。

3. Ⅱ、Ⅲ和aVF导联ST段位于等电位线。T波在Ⅱ导联低平，在Ⅲ和aVF导联倒置。

心电图诊断与解析

诊断：窦性心律；陈旧性下壁心肌梗死。

解析：在痊愈过程中，梗死部位的瘢痕组织可以收缩。部位局限的心肌梗死，如下壁心肌梗死，由于瘢痕组织收缩，无电活性区域缩小，心电图上的Q波振幅降低或消失。此心电图中，Ⅲ和aVF导联有病理性Q波，仅Ⅲ导联的Q波显而可见（见图34-1），诊断可能被遗漏。因此在心电图诊断中，应仔细观察每个导联中的每个波和段。

3. ST segments close to the isoelectric line in leads Ⅱ, Ⅲ and aVF. T waves are low in lead Ⅱ and inverted in leads Ⅲ and aVF.

ECG Interpretation

Sinus rhythm, old inferior myocardial infarction.

The scar tissue of the infarction may contract during the healing process. With limited myocardial infarction, such as inferior infarction, scar tissue contraction may cause the size of area without electrically viability to decrease, leading to a decrease in Q wave amplitude or disappearance. In this ECG, there is pathological Q wave in leads Ⅲ and aVF, but only Q wave in lead Ⅲ is easily distinguishable (see Fig. 34-1), and thus the diagnosis may be missed. Therefore, when making a diagnosis in ECG, every wave and segment in all leads should be inspected carefully.

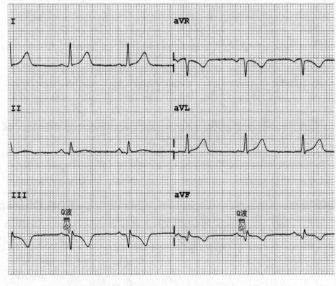

图34-1　病理性Q波

Fig. 34-1　Pathologic Q wave

图例35 陈旧性后侧壁心肌梗死

Case 35 Old Posterolateral Myocardial Infarction

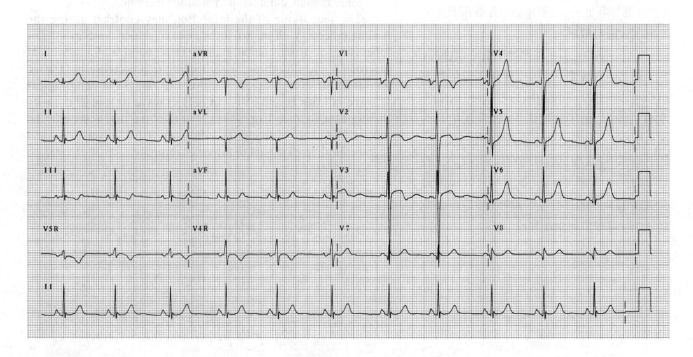

心电图特点

1. 心 率: 67次/min; PR间 期: 135 ms; QRS波时间: 88 ms; QT/QTc间期: 384/405 ms; QRS波电轴: 84°。

2. QRS波在V1导联呈Rs型, V7和V8导联呈qR型, aVL导联呈Qr型。ST段在所有

ECG Characteristics

1. HR: 67 bpm; PR: 135 ms; QRS D: 88 ms; QT/QTc: 384/405 ms; QRS Axis: 84°.

2. QRS complexes are Rs pattern in lead V1, qR pattern in leads V7 and V8, and Qr pattern in lead aVL. ST segments close to isoelectric line in all leads. T waves are inverted in lead V1, upright in leads I, V7, V8 and aVL. P–terminal force in lead V1 is >0.04 mm · s.

导联位于或接近等电位线。T波在V1导联倒置，Ⅰ、aVL和V7、V8导联直立。V1导联Ptf绝对值＞0.04 mm·s。

心电图诊断与解析

诊断：窦性心律；陈旧性后侧壁心肌梗死；左房肥大。

解析：如前所述（图例28），标准12导联心电图并不直接检测左心室后基底部和侧壁，推荐记录后壁附加导联。此心电图中，V1导联R波高大提示后壁心肌梗死，V7和V8导联有病理性Q波，从而肯定后壁心肌梗死（见图35-1）。aVL导联有病理性Q波，提示梗死累及至侧壁。

ECG Interpretation

Sinus rhythm, old posterolateral myocardial infarction, left atrial enlargement.

As mentioned before (see case 28), the standard 12-lead ECG does not directly examine the posterior basal and lateral areas of the left ventricle and use of additional posterior leads is recommended. In this ECG, dominant R wave in lead V1 suggests and pathological Q wave in additional leads V7 and V8 confirms posterior myocardial infarction (see Fig. 35-1). The presence of pathological Q wave in lead aVL suggests the infarction may have been extended to lateral area of the left ventricle.

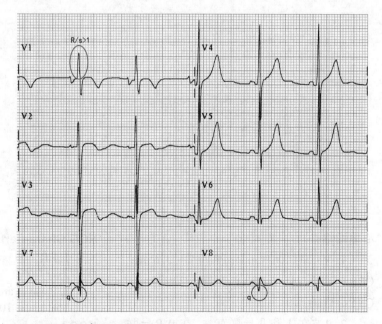

图35-1　R波高大和病理性Q波

Fig. 35-1　Dominant R wave and pathological Q wave

图例36 窦性心动过速

Case 36 Sinus Tachycardia

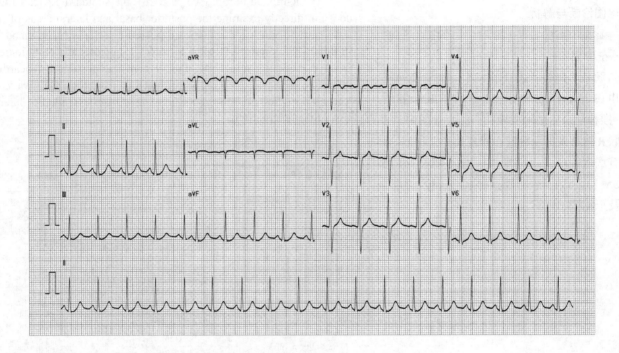

心电图特点

1. 心率：106次/min；PR间期：126 ms；QRS波时间：78 ms；QT/QTc间期：322/427 ms；QRS波电轴：70°。

2. P波在 I 和 II 导联直立，在aVR导联倒置。心率＞100次/min。

ECG Characteristics

1. HR: 106 bpm; PR: 126 ms; QRS D: 78 ms; QT/QTc: 322/427 ms; QRS axis: 70°.

2. P waves are upright in leads I and II , and inverted in lead aVR.

3. HR is ＞ 100 bpm.

ECG Interpretation

Sinus tachycardia.

心电图诊断与解析

诊断：窦性心动过速。

解析：分析心电图的第一步是判断主导心律。阅读心电图首先是观察或寻找P波。正常窦性心律，P波在Ⅰ和Ⅱ导联直立的，在aVR导联倒置。任何其他窦房结以外的心律称为"异位心律"。然后是计算心率，心率=60 s/PP（或RR）间期。这种计算心率的方法并不容易和快速，还有比较便捷的心率估计方法（详见图例37）。在成人，窦性心律大于100次/min，定义为窦性心动过速。此心电图中，P波在Ⅰ和Ⅱ导联直立的，在aVR导联倒置，表示心律来自窦房结，心率大于100次/min（见图36-1），因此心电图诊断为窦性心动过速。

The first step of the ECG interpretation is to determine the dominant rhythm. The first thing is to look or to find the P wave when reading an ECG. In normal sinus rhythm, the P waves are upright in leads Ⅰ and Ⅱ and inverted in lead aVR. Any other rhythm beyond the sinus node is called "ectopic rhythm". The second step is to calculate the heart rate. The heart rate is = 60 s / PP interval or RR interval. However, using this formula is not easy and quick, there is a more efficient way to estimate the heart rate (for details, see case 37). In adults, sinus rhythm with a rate greater than 100 bpm is defined as sinus tachycardia. In this ECG, the P waves are upright in leads Ⅰ and Ⅱ and inverted in lead aVR, indicate the rhythm is from sinus node; the rate is above 100 bpm (see Fig. 36-1). Therefore the ECG interpretation is sinus tachycardia.

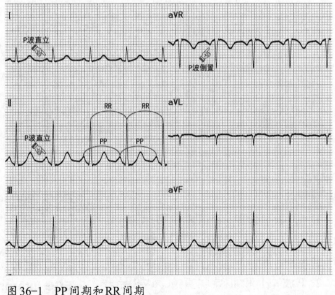

图36-1　PP间期和RR间期

Fig. 36-1　PP interval and RR interval

图例37　窦性心动过速

Case 37　Sinus Tachycardia

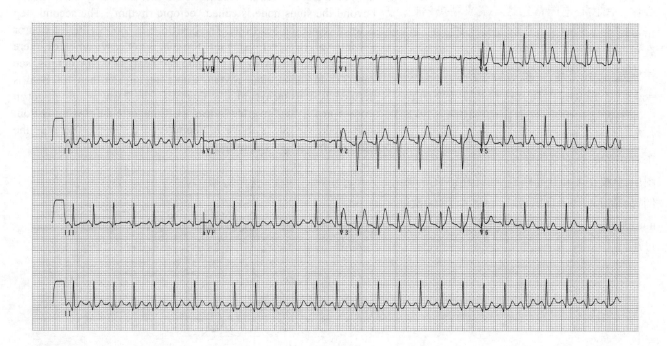

心电图特点

1. 心 率：162次/min；PR间 期：120 ms；QRS波时间：70 ms；QT/QTc间期：240/394 ms；QRS波电轴：79°。

2. P波：Ⅰ和Ⅱ导联直立，aVR导联倒置。心率＞100次/min。

ECG Characteristics

1. HR: 162 bpm; PR: 120 ms; QRS D: 70 ms; QT/QTc: 240/394 ms; QRS axis: 79°.

2. P waves are upright in leads Ⅰ and Ⅱ, and inverted in lead aVR. HR is > 100 bpm.

ECG Interpretation

Sinus tachycardia.

心电图诊断与解析

诊断：窦性心动过速。

解析：窦性心动过速是窦性冲动形成异常所致的心律失常。通常窦性心动过速发作时的心率小于150次/min，但有时也可高达150次/min以上，尤其是青少年和儿童。此心电图是一例23岁发热的患者，心率大于150次/min。有两种方法可计算或估计心率。第一种方法，标准的心电图走纸速度是25 mm/min，垂直的线可以用来测量时间。两粗线，也就是一大格或5小格，是0.20 s。数30大格（6 s）中P波或QRS波数，乘以10，就是心率。第二种方法，如图37-1所示，假如两个P波或QRS波间隔1大格，心率是300次/min，间隔2大格，心率是150次/min，间隔3大格，心率是100次/min，等等。记忆这些简单的数字，心率可以用目测来估计。

The sinus tachycardia is arrhythmia of sinus impulse formation. Usually the heart rate is below 150 bpm during the tachycardia episode, but sometimes the rate may be higher than 150 bpm, especially in teenagers and children. This ECG is an example of 23-year old case with fever, the heart rate is above 150 bpm. Two methods can be used to calculate or estimate the heart rate. First, the ECG paper moves at a standardized 25 mm/s and the vertical lines can be used to measure time. Each interval between 2 thicker lines (in other words, a large squre or 5 small squares) represents 0.20 s. Therefore, counting the number of the P waves or QRS complexes within 30 large squares (6 seconds) and multiplying it by 10 will yield the heart rate. Second, when two P waves or QRS complexes is one large square apart the rate is 300 bmp, two large squares apart the rate is 150 bmp, and three large squares apart the rate is 100 bmp, etc (see Fig. 37-1). Memorizing these simple numbers can help estimate the heart rate at a glance.

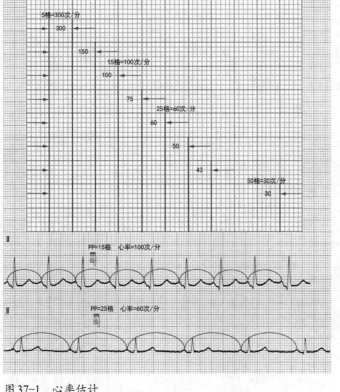

图37-1　心率估计

Fig. 37-1　Estimation of heart rate

图例38 窦性心动过缓

Case 38 Sinus Bradycardia

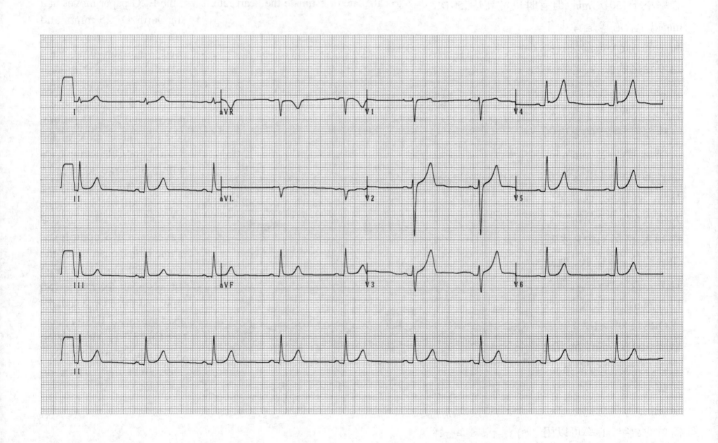

心电图特点

1. 心率: 53次/min; PR间期: 160 ms; QRS波时间: 94 ms; QT/QTc间期: 426/399 ms; QRS波电轴: 83°。

2. P波: Ⅰ和Ⅱ导联直立, aVR导联倒置。心率 < 60次/min。

心电图诊断与解析

诊断: 窦性心动过缓。

解析: 正常窦性心律, 静息心率低于60次/min, 定义为心动过缓。此心电图中, P波在Ⅰ和Ⅱ导联直立, 在aVR导联倒置, 表示心律来自窦房结, 心率低于60次/min(见图38-1), 因此此心电图诊断为窦性心动过缓。窦性心动过缓是窦性冲动形成异常所致的心律失常。运用前面所述的方法(图例37), 两个P波间隔接近6大格, 能目测估计心率约为50次/min。

ECG Characteristics

1. HR: 53 bpm; PR: 160 ms; QRS D: 94 ms; QT/QTc: 426/399 ms; QRS axis: 83°.

2. P waves are upright in leads Ⅰ and Ⅱ, and inverted in lead aVR. HR is < 60 bpm.

ECG Interpretation

Sinus bradycardia.

In normal sinus rhythm, a resting heart rate below 60 bpm is defined as bradycardia. In this ECG, the P waves are upright in leads Ⅰ and Ⅱ and inverted in lead aVR, indicate the rhythm is from sinus node, the rate is below 60 bpm (see Fig. 38–1), so the interpretation is sinus bradycardia. The sinus bradycardia is arrhythmia of sinus impulse formation. Using the method described before (case 37), close to 6 larger squares between two P waves, the heart rate can be estimated about 50 bmp at a glance.

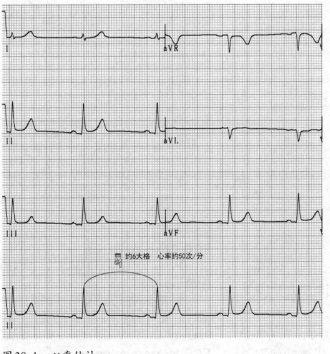

约6大格　心率约50次/分

图38-1　心率估计

Fig. 38-1　Estimation of heart rate

图例39　窦性心律不齐

Case 39　Sinus Arrhythmia

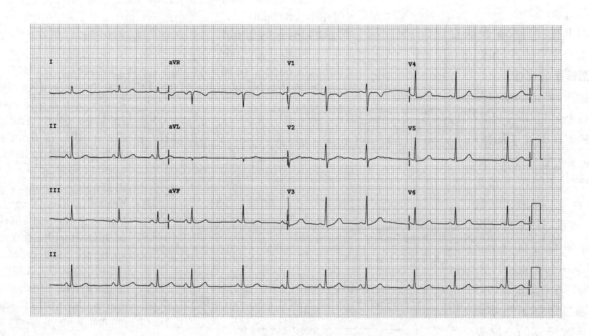

心电图特点

1. 心 率：68次/min；PR间 期：152 ms；QRS波时间：75 ms；QT/QTc间期：392/417 ms；QRS波电轴：67°。

2. P波在Ⅰ和Ⅱ导联直立，在aVR导联倒置。P波相同，同一导联上PP间期差异 > 120 ms。

ECG Characteristics

1. HR: 68 bpm; PR: 152 ms; QRS D: 75 ms; QT/QTc: 392/417 ms; QRS axis: 67°.

2. P waves are upright in leads Ⅰ and Ⅱ, and inverted in lead aVR. The P waves are similar and the differences between PP intervals are > 120 ms at the same lead.

ECG Interpretation

Sinus arrhythmia.

心电图诊断与解析

诊断：窦性心律不齐。

解析：窦性心律通常是规则的，但有时也可以不规则。若在同一导联中，PP间期之间的差异大于120 ms，定为窦性心律不齐。心率变化常发生在呼吸运动中，称之为呼吸性窦性心律不齐。吸气时心率增快，呼气时心率减慢，常见于儿童和青年人。假如非青年人，不发生在呼吸运动中，常可伴有心动过缓，可能是窦房结功能不全或病态窦房结综合征的征象。由于PP间期是不等的，推荐用数30大格中P波或QRS波数乘以10的方法来计算心率。如图39-1所示，此心电图Ⅱ导联节律图上，P波相同，PP间期差异 > 120 ms，诊断为窦性心律不齐。

Generally, the sinus rhythm is regular, but sometimes the rhythm may be irregular. If the differences between PP intervals are more than 120 ms at the same lead, the condition is defined as sinus arrhythmia. The heart rate often changes during breathing, which is called respiratory sinus arrhythmia. The heart rate increases with inspiration and decreases with expiration. It is common in children and young. If it is not in young and not occurring with breathing, then it often accompanies bradycardia, potentially it is a sign of sinus node dysfunction or sick sinus syndrome. Because the PP interval is different, the method counting the number of P waves or QRS complexes within 30 large squares and multiply by 10 is recommended to calculate the heart rate. In this ECG, P waves are similar and the differences between PP intervals are > 120 ms (see Fig. 39-1). The ECG interpretation is sinus arrhythmia.

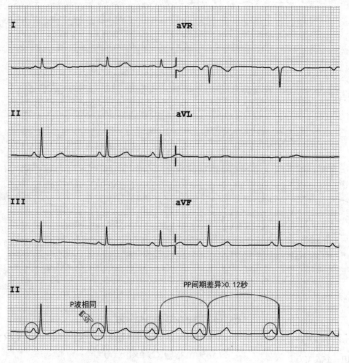

图39-1　PP间期差异

Fig. 39-1　Differences between PP intervals

图例 40　窦性心动过缓，窦性静止

Case 40　Sinus Bradycardia, Sinus Arrest

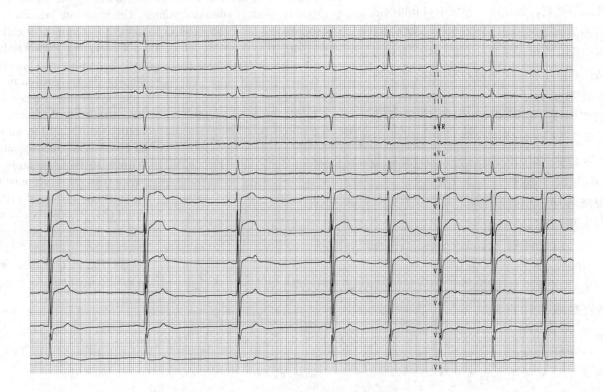

心电图特点

1. 心率: 31 ~ 59次/min; PR间期: 200 ms; QRS波时间: 110 ms; QT/QTc间期: 456/389 ms; QRS波电轴: 60°。

ECG Characteristics

1. HR: 31 ~ 59 bpm; PR: 200 ms; QRS D: 110 ms; QT/QTc: 456/389 ms; QRS axis: 60°.

2. P waves are upright in leads Ⅰ and Ⅱ, and inverted in lead aVR. The long PP intervals are not a multiple of the short PP

2. P波在Ⅰ和Ⅱ导联直立，在aVR导联倒置。长PP间期不是短PP间期的倍数。T波在V1～V5导联直立，有切迹。U波在V1～V3导联明显。

心电图诊断与解析

诊断：窦性心动过缓；窦性静止；T波改变；U波明显。

解析：正常时，窦房结产生冲动来维持和调节稳定和正常的心率。窦性静止的定义是窦房结在一定时间内不产生冲动，在心电图上表现为无P、QRS和T波，长时间停顿，即长PP间期。窦性静止的时间是随机不等的，因此窦性静止的特点是长PP间期不是基础PP间期的倍数。长间期可以被窦性心动终止，或者被交界性或室性逸搏终止。此心电图上有三次长PP间期和五次短PP间期，长PP间期不是短PP间期的倍数（见图40-1）。在鉴别诊断上着重考虑窦性静止。

intervals. T waves are upright in leads V1 ~ V5 with notches. U waves are prominent upright in leads V1 ~ V3.

ECG Interpretation

Sinus bradycardia, sinus arrest, T wave abnormalities, U wave abnormalities.

Normally the sinus node generates the impulse to maintain and regulate a steady and normal heart rate. Sinus arrest is defined as a failure of impulse formation in the sinus node for certain period of time. It is manifested by the absence of the P wave and QRS-T complex, a long pause (long PP interval) in ECG. Because the duration of sinus arrest is random and variable, so the distinguishing feature of sinus arrest is that the long PP interval is not a multiple of the short (basic) PP interval. The pause may be terminated by sinus beat or A-V junctional or ventricular escape beat. In this ECG, there are three long PP intervals and five short PP intervals. The long PP intervals are not a multiple of the short PP intervals (see Fig. 40-1). Sinus arrest should be considered high on the differential diagnosis.

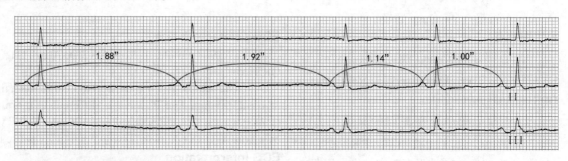

图40-1　长PP间期与短PP间期不成倍数

Fig. 40-1　Long PP intervals are not a multiple of the short PP intervals

图例41　房性期前收缩

- -

Case 41　Atrial Premature Complex

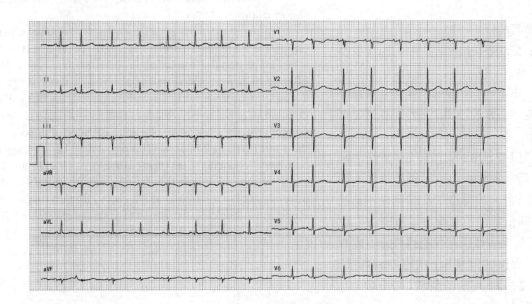

心电图特点

1. 心 率: 98次/min; PR间 期: 148 ms; QRS波时间: 70 ms; QT/QTc间期: 358/455 ms; QRS波电轴: −6°。

2. 基本节律中出现提前的异位P(P′)波; P′波形态与窦性P波不同。P′R间期 > 120 ms。P′波后QRS波形态正常。代偿间期不完全。

ECG Characteristics

1. HR: 98 bpm; PR: 148 ms; QRS D: 70 ms; QT/QTc: 358/455 ms; QRS axis: −6°.

2. The ectopic P (P′) wave appears earlier than the cardiac cycles of basic rhythm. The P′ wave is different in morphology from the sinus P waves. The P′R interval is > 120 ms. The P′ wave is followed by a normal QRS complex. The compensatory pause is incomplete.

ECG Interpretation

Sinus rhythm, atrial premature complex.

心电图诊断与解析

诊断：窦性心律；房性期前收缩。

解析：房性期前收缩是一种常见的心律失常，起源于窦房结以外的心房。由于期前收缩起源窦房结以外，异位P（P′）的形态与窦性P波不同。通常心房激动经房室结下传心室，P′R间期＞120 ms，并形成形态正常的（窄的）QRS波。代偿间期是期前收缩前的P波和期前收缩后的P波之间的间期，若这代偿间期等于2倍基本PP间期，代偿间期完全，若小于2倍，代偿间期不完全。房性期前收缩通常代偿间期不完全，原因是期前收缩进入窦房结，重整其节律，其后的P波提前出现（见图41-1）。此心电图上有一个期前收缩，其特点符合所有房性期前收缩的特点（见图41-2）。

Atrial premature complex (APC) is a common arrhythmia originating in the atria outside the sinus node. Since the premature beat initiates outside the sinus node, the ectopic P (P′) wave appears different morphology from those seen in normal sinus rhythm. Typically, the atrial impulse propagates normally through the A–V node and into the ventricles, resulting in P′R interval > 120 ms and normal (narrow) QRS complex. The interval between the P wave preceding the premature beat and following the premature beat is the compensatory pause. The compensatory pause is considered complete or full if it equals two of the basic PP interval. The pause is considered incomplete or not full if it is less than two of the basic PP interval. The APC usually has an incomplete compensatory pause, because the premature beat usually enters the sinus node and resets its timing, causing the next sinus P to appear earlier than expected (see Fig. 41-1). In this ECG, there are three premature beats that meet all of the characteristics of APC (see Fig. 41-2).

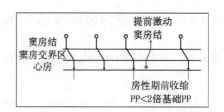

图 41-1　代偿间期不完全

Fig. 41-1　Incomplete compensatory pause

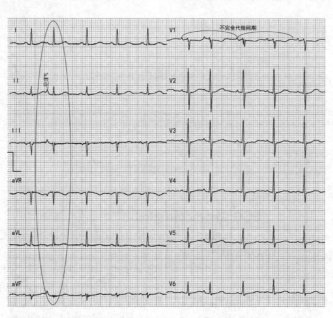

图 41-2　房性期前收缩

Fig. 41-2　Atrial premature complex

图例42 房性期前收缩伴心室内差异传导

Case 42 Atrial Premature Complex with Aberrant Intraventricular Conduction

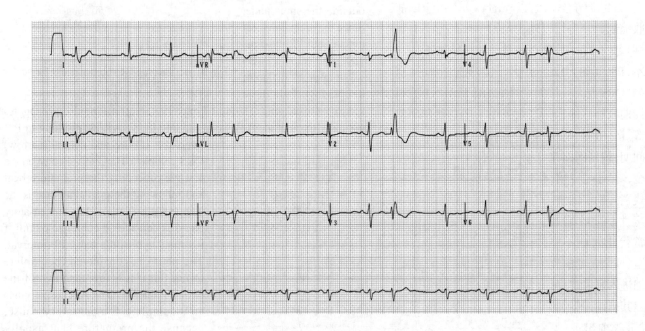

心电图特点

1. 心 率: 76次/min; PR间 期: 146 ms; QRS波时间: 84 ms; QT/QTc间期: 392/450 ms; QRS波电轴: −38°。

2. 基本节律中出现提前的P′波; P′波形态与窦性P波不同。P′R间期 > 120 ms。P′波后QRS波增宽畸形。代偿间期不完全。

ECG Characteristics

1. HR: 76 bpm; PR: 146 ms; QRS D: 84 ms; QT/QTc: 392/450 ms; QRS axis: −38°.

2. The P′ waves appear earlier than the cardiac cycle of basic rhythm. The P′ waves are different in morphology from the sinus P waves. The P′R intervals are > 120 ms. The P′ waves are followed by QRS complexes with wide and abnormal morphology. The compensatory pauses are incomplete.

心电图诊断与解析

诊断：窦性心律；房性期前收缩伴心室内差异传导；电轴左偏。

解析：有时，提前的心房激动进入心室时，遇到一处或多处心室内传导分支或束支仍处于不应期。激动在处于不应期的心室中传导，传导速度降低或传导中断，产生宽大畸形的QRS波，称为心室内差异传导。右束支的不应期通常长于左束支，因此QRS波畸形常呈右束支阻滞图形（V1导联呈rsR′型，见图例89）。此时，房性期前收缩伴心室内差异传导应与室性期前收缩相鉴别，P′波和代偿间期不完全将有助于鉴别诊断。此心电图上，在V1导联上能清楚发现QRS波宽大畸形，呈rsR′型，提早的P′波和代偿间期不完全，所有这些支持房性期前收缩伴心室内差异传导（见图42-1）。

ECG Interpretation

Sinus rhythm, atrial premature complex with aberrant intraventricular conduction, left axis deviation.

Sometimes, the premature atrial impulse propagates into the ventricles and finds one or more of the conducting fascicles or bundle branches still in refractory period. When the impulse traverses the ventricles during a refractory period, the conduction is reduced in speed or blocked, thus QRS complex with wide and abnormal morphology occurs, this condition is called aberrant intraventricular conduction. The refractory period of right bundle branch usually lasts longer than that of left bundle branch, so the abnormal QRS complex often occurs in right bundle branch block pattern (rsR′ pattern in lead V1, see case 89). In this situation, one should make differential diagnosis between APC and ventricular premature complex (VPC). The P′ wave and incomplete compensatory pause are helpful for making differential diagnosis. In this ECG, wide and abnormal morphology QRS complex in rsR′ pattern can be seen clearly in lead V1, earlier P′ waves and incomplete compensatory pauses, all of those suggest APC with aberrant intraventricular conduction (see Fig. 42-1).

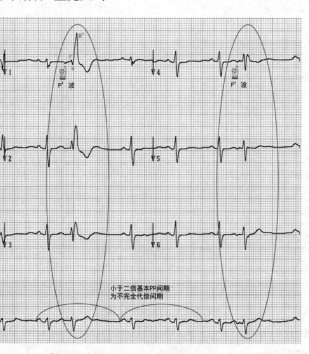

图42-1　房性期前收缩伴心室内差异传导

Fig. 42-1　Atrial premature complex with aberrant intraventricular conduction

图例43　房性期前收缩未下传

Case 43　Non-conducted (Blocked) Atrial Premature Complex

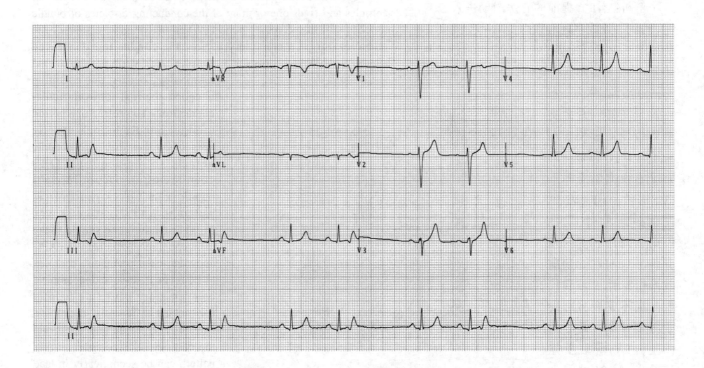

心电图特点

1. 心 率：71次/min；PR间 期：184 ms；QRS波时间：80 ms；QT/QTc间期：382/417 ms；QRS波电轴：76°。

2. 基本节律中出现提前的P′波；P′波形

ECG Characteristics

1. HR: 71 bpm; PR: 184 ms; QRS D: 80 ms; QT/QTc: 382/417 ms; QRS axis: 76°.

2. The P′ waves appear earlier than the cardiac cycle of basic rhythm. The P′ waves are different in morphology from the sinus P waves. All P′ waves are not followed by QRS complexes. The

态与窦性P波不同。P'波后无QRS波。代偿间期不完全。

心电图诊断与解析

诊断：窦性心律；房性期前收缩未下传。

解析：有时，提前的激动遇到房室结的不应期，过早的房性期前收缩不能下传心室，这类期前收缩称为房性期前收缩未下传或阻滞型房性期前收缩。在心电图上，房性期前收缩未下传表现为P'波后无QRS波，形成一长间期。此时房性期前收缩未下传应与窦性静止或窦房阻滞相鉴别。在长RR间期中寻找P'波，将有助鉴别诊断。此心电图上，所有的P'后均无QRS波，P'波融入前ST段中，但清晰可见，代偿间期不完全，支持心电图诊断为房性期前收缩未下传（见图43-1）。

compensatory pauses are incomplete.

ECG Interpretation

Sinus rhythm, non-conducted (blocked) atrial premature complex.

Sometimes, an early atrial premature complex may not be conducted to the ventricles, as the premature beat reaches to A-V node when it is still in refractory. Such P' wave is called non-conducted or blocked APC. In ECG, non-conducted APC presents that the P' wave is not followed by a QRS complex, leading to a long pause. In this situation, a differential diagnosis should be made between APC and sinus arrest or sinoatrial block. Finding P' wave within the long pause will be helpful for make the differentiation. In this ECG, all P' waves are not followed by QRS complexes, and P' waves are merged into the preceding ST segments yet clearly distinguishable. The compensatory pauses are incomplete. These suggest that the ECG interpretation is non-conducted APC (see Fig. 43-1).

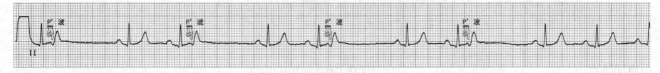

图 43-1　房性期前收缩未下传

Fig. 43-1　Nonconducted atrial premature complex

图例44 房性期前收缩

Case 44 Atrial Premature Complex

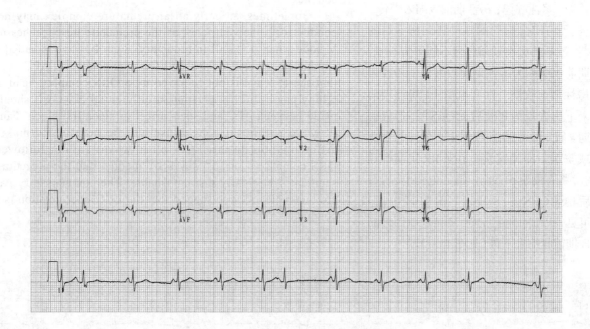

心电图特点

    1. 心率: 67次/min; PR间期: 124 ms; QRS波时间: 82 ms; QT/QTc间期: 410/433 ms; QRS波电轴: 25°。

    2. 基本节律中出现提前的P′波; P′波形态与窦性P波不同。P′R间期>120 ms。P′波后QRS波增宽畸形或正常或无QRS波。代

ECG Characteristics

    1. HR: 67 bpm; PR: 124 ms; QRS D: 82 ms; QT/QTc: 410/433 ms; QRS axis: 25°.

    2. The P′ waves appear earlier than the cardiac cycle of the basic rhythm. The P′ waves are different in morphology from the sinus P waves.The P′R intervals are > 120 ms.The P′ waves are followed by a QRS complex with wide and abnormal morphology or a normal QRS complex or not followed by a QRS complex. The compensatory

偿间期不完全。

心电图诊断与解析

诊断：窦性心律；房性期前收缩；房性期前收缩伴心室内差异传导；房性期前收缩未下传。

解析：如前所述（图例41～43），房性期前收缩有三种不同的表现。第一种是传导正常，在心电图上QRS波与其他QRS波相似。第二种是心室内差异传导，在心电图上QRS波宽大畸形。第三种是未下传，在心电图上P′波后无QRS波。此心电图上，房性期前收缩的三种不同表现都存在（见图44-1）。房性期前收缩传导不同，取决于提早的程度和前心动周期长度。前者越早或后者越长，越容易发生心室内差异传导或未下传。

pauses are incomplete.

ECG Interpretation

Sinus rhythm, atrial premature complex, atrial premature complex with aberrant intraventricular conduction, nonconduction atrial premature complex.

As mentioned before (case 41～43), APC may be conducted to the ventricles in three different ways. The first way is normal conduction, which leads to similar QRS complex to the others in the ECG. The second way is to be conducted with aberration, which leads to wide QRS complex of abnormal morphology. The third way is to be non-conducted or blocked, where the P′ wave is not followed by a QRS complex. In this ECG, all three different outcomes are present (see Fig. 44-1). The outcome of APC conduction depends on the degree of prematurity and the preceding cycle length. The former is earlier or the later is longer, the more likely for aberration or non-conduction to occur.

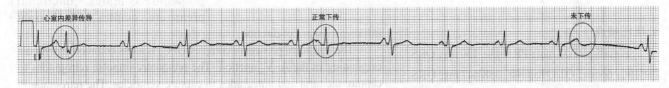

图44-1　房性期前收缩向心室传导的三种不同类型

Fig. 44-1　Three different ways in atrial premature complex conducted to the ventricles

图例45　交界性期前收缩伴心室内差异传导

Case 45　Junctional Premature Complex with Aberrant Intraventricular Conduction

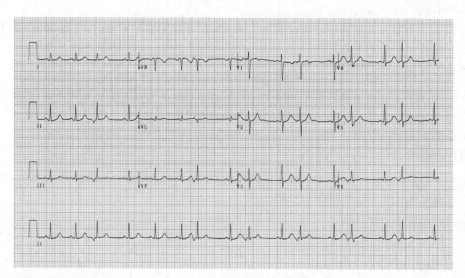

ECG Characteristics

1. HR: 94 bpm; PR: 130 ms; QRS D: 66 ms; QT/QTc: 358/447 ms; QRS axis: 59°.

2. The P′ waves appear earlier than the cardiac cycles of the basic rhythm. The P′ waves are inverted in lead II. The P′ R intervals are < 120 ms. The P′ waves are followed by normal or wide QRS complexes. The compensatory pauses are complete or incomplete.

ECG Interpretation

Sinus rhythm, junctional premature complex, junctional premature complex with aberrant intraventricular conduction.

The junctional premature complex (JPC) is a less common arrhythmia originating in the A–V junction. The premature impulse retrogrades to capture the atria and antegrades to capture ventricles. The retrograde P′ wave is usually inverted in leads II and upright in lead aVR. The P′ wave may precede, superimpose on, or follow the QRS complex, which depends upon the location of the ectopic focus in the A–V junction and the state of the antegrade and retrograde conduction system (see Fig. 45–1). If the P′ wave precedes the QRS complex, the P′ R interval will be < 120 ms. If the P′ wave comes after the QRS complex, the RP′ interval will be < 200 ms. In most instances, the morphology of the QRS complex is normal. Abnormal

心电图特点

1. 心率: 94次/min; PR间期: 130 ms; QRS波时间: 66 ms; QT/QTc间期: 358/447 ms; QRS波电轴: 59°。

2. 基本节律中出现提前的P′波; P′在II导联中倒置。P′R间期<120 ms。P′波后QRS波正常或宽大畸形。代偿间期完全或不完全。

心电图诊断与解析

诊断: 窦性心律; 交界性期前收缩; 交

界性期前收缩伴心室内差异传导。

　　解析：交界性期前收缩是不常见的心律失常，起源于房室交界区。提前的冲动逆传夺获心房，前传夺获心室。逆行P′波通常在Ⅱ导联中倒置，在aVR导联中直立。P′波可以在QRS波前，或重叠在QRS波上，或在QRS波后，取决于异位节律点的部位，逆传和前传系统的状态（见图45-1）。假如P′波在QRS波前，P′R间期<120 ms。假如P′波在QRS波后，RP′间期<200 ms。在大多数情况下，QRS波形态正常。假如存在心室内差异传导，QRS波畸形。假如前传阻滞，P′波后无QRS波。由于期前收缩不能进入窦房结，重整其节律，因此通常代偿间期完全，但有时也可不完全。此心电图上有六次期前收缩，P′波均在QRS波前，P′R<120 ms，符合交界性期前收缩的特点（见图45-2）。

QRS complex may be seen if there is aberrant intraventricular conduction. If antegrade is blocked, the P′ wave will not follow the QRS complex. Usually, the compensatory pause is complete, as JPC usually does not enter the sinus node and reset its timing. But sometimes it can be incomplete. In this ECG, there are six premature beats, all P′ waves precede the QRS complexes and the P′R intervals are < 120 ms (see Fig. 45-2), which follow the characteristics of JPC.

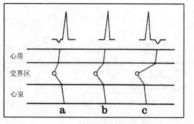

图45-1　P′波与QRS波的关系

Fig. 45-1　P′ wave and QRS complex

注：　a. 逆传快于前传：P′波在QRS波前；b. 逆传与前传相等：P′波重叠在在QRS波上；c. 逆传慢于前传：P′波在QRS波后

Notes：a. Retrogrades earlier than antegrades：the P′wave precedes the QRS complex;b. Retrogrades equal to antegrades：the P′ wave superimposes on the QRS complex;c. Retrogrades later than antegrades：the P′ wave follows the QRS complex

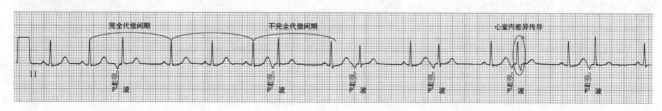

图45-2　交界性期前收缩

Fig. 45-2　Junctional premature complex

图例 46　交界性期前收缩

Case 46　Junctional Premature Complex

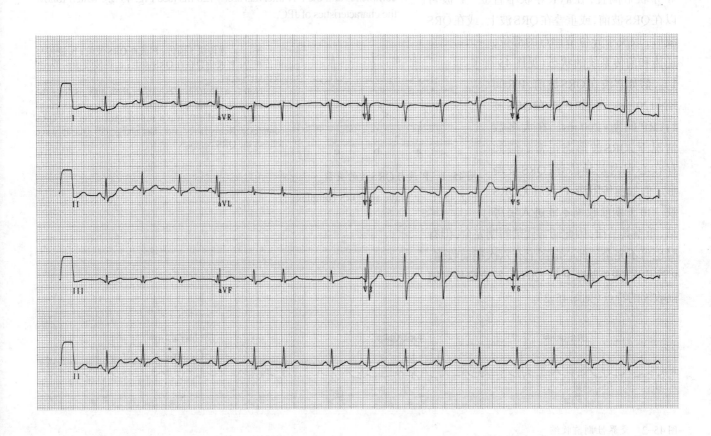

心电图特点

1. 心率：95次/min；PR间期：124 ms；QRS波时间：92 ms；QT/QTc间期：354/444 ms；QRS波电轴：37°。

2. 基本节律中出现提前的QRS波，其前后无P′波。代偿间期完全。

心电图诊断与解析

诊断：窦性心律；交界性期前收缩。

解析：此心电图上，提早的QRS波形态正常，代偿间期完全，符合交界性期前收缩的特点（见图46-1）。问题是为何QRS波前后无P′波。有两种解释：其一是当逆传和前传相等，P′波重叠在QRS波中，不能清晰可见；其二是逆传阻滞，未夺获心房，在心电图上无P′波。

ECG Characteristics

1. HR: 95 bpm; PR: 124 ms; QRS D: 92 ms; QT/QTc: 354/444 ms; QRS axis: 37°.

2. The QRS complex appears earlier than the cardiac cycle of the basic rhythm. There is no P′ wave before or after the QRS complex.

3. The compensatory pause is complete.

ECG Interpretation

Sinus rhythm, junctional premature complex.

In this ECG, the premature QRS complex is normal and the compensatory pause is complete, which follow the characteristics of JPC (see Fig. 46-1). The question is why there is no P′ wave before or after the QRS complex. There are two reasons. One is that the P′ wave cannot be seen clearly because the P′ wave superimposes on the QRS complex when retrograde is equal to antegrade. Other is that retrograde is blocked and does not capture the atria resulting in no P′ wave in ECG.

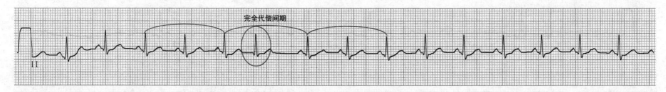

图46-1　交界性期前收缩

Fig. 46-1　Junctional premature complex

图例47　交界性期前收缩伴心室内差异传导

Case 47　Junctional Premature Complex with Aberrant Intraventricular Conduction

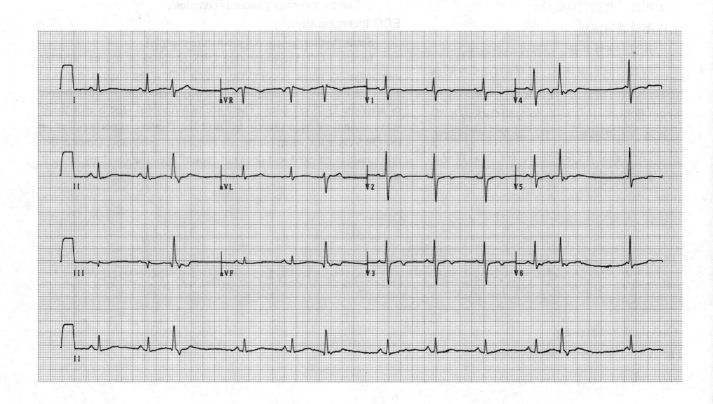

心电图特点

1. 心率：73次/min；PR间期：144 ms；QRS波时间：84 ms；QT/QTc间期：388/427 ms；QRS波电轴：29°。

2. 基本节律中出现提前的宽QRS波。P′波在QRS波后，在Ⅱ导联中倒置。RP′间期<200 ms。代偿间期完全。

心电图诊断与解析

诊断：窦性心律；交界性期前收缩。

解析：此心电图上有3次提早的宽QRS波，其后有P′波，Ⅱ导联中P′波倒置。RP′间期<200 ms，代偿间期完全。根据以上特点，鉴别诊断上着重考虑交界性期前收缩伴心室内差异传导（见图47-1）。

ECG Characteristics

1. HR: 73 bpm; PR: 144 ms; QRS D: 84 ms; QT/QTc: 388/427 ms; QRS axis: 29°.

2. The wide QRS complexes appear earlier than the cardiac cycle of the basic rhythm.The P′ waves are after the QRS complexes and inverted in lead Ⅱ. The RP′ intervals are < 200 ms. The compensatory pauses are complete.

ECG Interpretation

Sinus rhythm, junctional premature complex with aberrant intraventricular conduction.

In this ECG, there are three wide and premature QRS complexes. The P′ waves occur after the QRS complexes and are inverted in lead Ⅱ. The RP′ intervals are < 200 ms and the compensatory pauses are complete. According to these characteristics, JPC with aberrant intraventricular conduction should be considered highly in differential diagnosis (see Fig. 47-1).

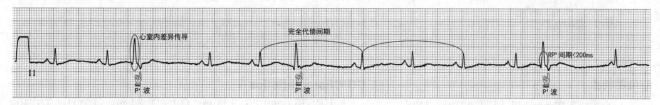

图 47-1 交界性期前收缩

Fig. 47-1 Junctional premature complex

图例48 室性期前收缩

Case 48 Ventricular Premature Complex

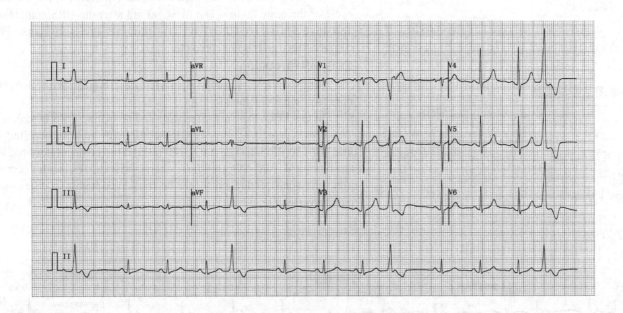

心电图特点

1. 心率: 76次/min; PR间期: 138 ms; QRS波时间: 84 ms; QT/QTc间期: 370/404 ms; QRS波电轴: 50°。

2. 提前出现宽大畸形的QRS波,前无P′波。

3. 期前收缩间期中窦性P波清晰可见,位于QRS波后。代偿间期完全。

ECG Characteristics

1. HR: 76 bpm; PR: 138 ms; QRS D: 84 ms; QT/QTc: 370/404 ms; QRS axis: 50°.

2. The wide QRS complexes with abnormal morphology appear prematurely without a preceding P′ waves.

3. The sinus P waves can be clearly identified after the QRS complexes. The compensatory pauses are complete.

ECG Interpretation

Sinus rhythm, ventricular premature complex.

心电图诊断与解析

诊断：窦性心律；室性期前收缩。

解析：室性期前收缩是起源于心室的一种常见的心律失常。在心电图上室性期前收缩的表现是提前出现宽大畸形的QRS波，其前无异位P(P′)波。QRS波时间常大于120 ms。由于室性期前收缩不能进入窦房结，不能重整窦房结的节律，因此通常代偿间期完全。在大多数情况下，在室性期前收缩中，窦性P波不能到达心室，因为心室仍处于室性期前收缩所产生的不应期中，这一现象称为房室分离。室性期前收缩中的P波，常被室性期前收缩的QRS波或T波所掩盖，不能清晰可见。但是有时，心电图中P波能清晰可见（见图48-1）。此心电图，提前出现宽大畸形的QRS波，前无P′波，清晰可见窦性P波在QRS波后（房室分离），以及代偿间期完全，所有这些特点提示心电图诊断是室性期前收缩。

Ventricular premature complex.

(VPC) is a common arrhythmia originating in ventricles. In ECG, VPC is present as a premature wide QRS complex with a different morphology from that of the sinus beat and without a preceding ectopic P (P′) wave. Often, the QRS duration is 120 ms or more. Usually the compensatory pause is complete because VPC does not enter the sinus node and interrupt the sinus node timing. In most instances, during the period of VPC, the sinus P wave cannot reach the ventricles as they are still refractory from the VPC. This phenomenon is called A–V dissociation. The P wave during the VPC cannot be clearly identified because it is masked by the QRS complex or T wave of the VPC. However, sometimes the P wave can be clearly identified as in this ECG (see Fig. 48–1). In this ECG, the wide QRS complexes of abnormal morphology appear prematurely without a preceding P′ wave, the sinus P waves can be clearly identified after the QRS complexes (A–V dissociation) and the compensatory pauses are complete, all of which suggest that the ECG interpretation should be VPC.

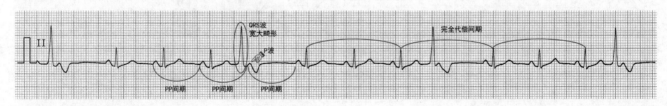

图48-1　室性期前收缩

Fig. 48–1　Ventricular premature complex

图例49　室性期前收缩

Case 49　Ventricular Premature Complex

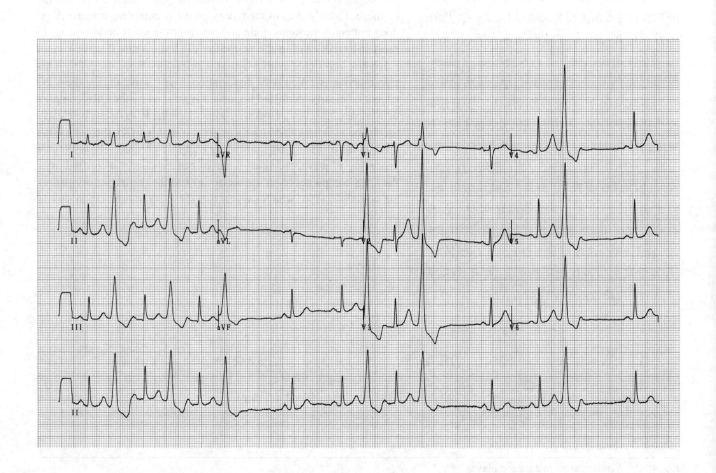

心电图特点

1. 心率：74次/min；PR间期：154 ms；QRS波时间：76 ms；QT/QTc间期：378/412 ms；QRS波电轴：75°。

2. 提前出现宽大畸形的QRS波，前无P′波。

3. 代偿间期完全或无代偿间期。

心电图诊断与解析

诊断：窦性心律；室性期前收缩。

解析：假如室性期前收缩较早出现，并不能阻止其后窦性P波的下传，室性期前收缩可以夹在两个正常窦性心动之间，而无代偿间期。这类室性期前收缩称为插入性室性期前收缩。此心电图上，共有三个插入性室性期前收缩（见图49-1）。

ECG Characteristics

1. HR: 74 bpm; PR: 154 ms; QRS D: 76 ms; QT/QTc: 378/412 ms; QRS axis: 75°.

2. The wide and abnormal morphology QRS complexes appear prematurely without a preceding P′ waves.

3. The compensatory pauses are complete or absent.

ECG Interpretation

Sinus rhythm, ventricular premature complex.

If a VPC occurs early enough, it will not prevent the conduction of the P wave that follows. The VPC then appears to be sandwiched between two normal sinus beats without a compensatory pause. This type of VPC is called an interpolated VPC. In this ECG, there are three interpolated VPCs (see Fig. 49-1).

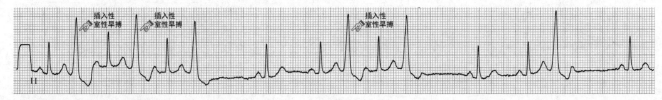

图 49-1　插入性室性期前收缩

Fig. 49-1　Interpolated ventricular premature complex

图例50　多源性室性期前收缩

Case 50　Multifocal Ventricular Premature Complex

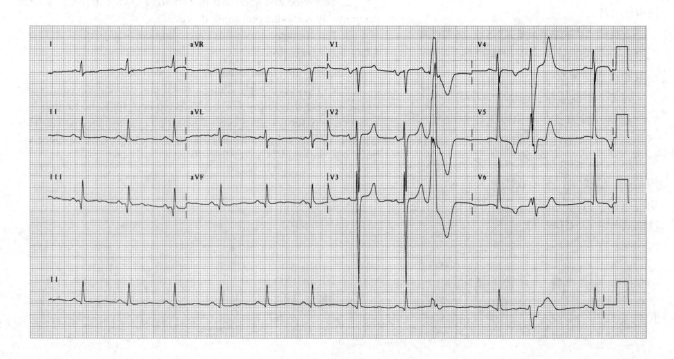

心电图特点

1. 心率：73次/min；PR间期：168 ms；QRS波时间：90 ms；QT/QTc间期：395/435 ms；QRS波电轴：62°。

2. 提前出现宽大畸形的QRS波，前无P′波。提前的QRS波形态和联律间期不同。代偿间

ECG Characteristics

1. HR: 73 bpm; PR: 168 ms; QRS D: 90 ms; QT/QTc: 395/435 ms; QRS axis: 62°.

2. The wide and abnormal morphology of QRS complexes appears prematurely without a preceding P′ waves. The morphologies and the coupling intervals of premature QRS complexes are different. The compensatory pauses are complete. P-terminal force in lead V1 is

期完全。V1 导联 Ptf 绝对值 > 0.04 mm · s。

3. V5 导联 R 波振幅 > 2.5 mV，$R_{V5}+S_{V1}$ > 3.5 mV，$R_{aVL}+S_{V3}$ > 2.8 mV。T 波在 Ⅱ、Ⅲ 和 aVF 导联低平，在 V4 ~ V6 导联倒置。V5 和 V6 导联 ST 段压低 ≥ 0.05 mV。

心电图诊断与解析

诊断：窦性心律；多源性室性期前收缩；左心房肥大；左心室肥大；ST-T 改变。

解析：室性期前收缩起源部位不同，QRS 波的形态不同。室性期前收缩可有单源和多源。单源室性期前收缩起源同一部位，在心电图上联律间期（与前 QRS 波之间的间期）恒定，QRS 波形态相同。多源室性期前收缩起源不同部位，在心电图上联律间期和 QRS 波形态常不同。此心电图上有两个期前收缩，联律间期和 QRS 波形态均不相同，表明室性期前收缩起源不同部位，为多源性室性期前收缩（见图 50-1）。

> 0.04 mm·s.

3. R wave in leads V5 is > 2.5 mV, $R_{V5} + S_{V1}$ > 3.5 mV, $R_{aVL} + S_{V3}$ > 2.8 mV. T waves are low and flat in leads Ⅱ, Ⅲ and aVF, and inverted in leads V4 ~ V6. ST segments depression in leads V5 and V6 is ≥ 0.05 mV.

ECG Interpretation

Sinus rhythm, multifocal ventricular premature complex, left atrial enlargement, left ventricular hypertrophy, ST-T abnormalities.

The QRS morphology of VPC varies according to its site of origin. VPCs can be either unifocal or multifocal. The unifocal VPCs have the same site of origin, resulting in similar coupling intervals (measured from the previous QRS complex) and the QRS morphologies may be the same in ECG. The multifocal VPCs have different sites of origin, and thus in ECG the coupling intervals and the QRS morphologies are usually different. In this ECG, there are two VPCs with different coupling intervals and the QRS morphologies, indicating different sites of origin, thus interpreted as multifocal VPCs (see Fig. 50-1).

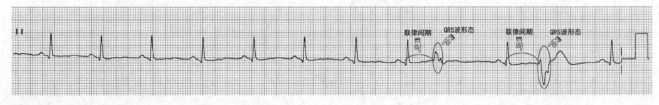

图 50-1 多源性室性期前收缩

Fig. 50-1 Multifocal ventricular premature complex

图例51 室性期前收缩二联律

Case 51 Bigeminal Ventricular Premature Complex

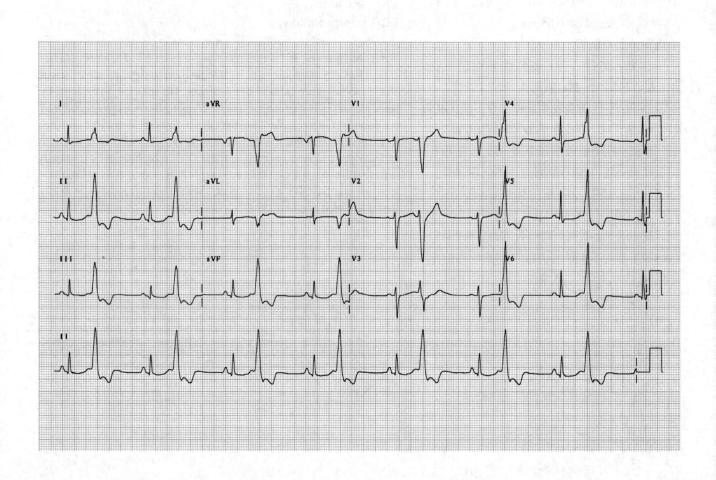

心电图特点

1. 心率: 86次/min; PR间期: 146 ms; QRS波时间: 90 ms; QT/QTc间期: 348/416 ms; QRS波电轴: 62°。

2. 提前出现宽大畸形的QRS波, 前无P'波。代偿间期完全。一个窦性QRS波跟随一个提前的QRS波。

心电图诊断与解析

诊断: 窦性心律; 室性期前收缩二联律。

解析: 期前收缩可以单个偶尔出现, 也可以特定的规律出现。二联律和三联律是描述特定规律的术语。期前收缩可以形成二联律, 连续出现一个窦性心动跟随一个期前收缩; 也可形成三联律, 连续出现两个窦性心动跟随一个期前收缩或一个窦性心动跟随两个期前收缩。此心电图, 一个窦性心动跟随一个室性期前收缩, 即室性期前收缩二联律(见图51-1)。

ECG Characteristics

1. HR: 86 bpm; PR: 146 ms; QRS D: 90 ms; QT/QTc: 348/416 ms; QRS axis: 62°.

2. The wide and abnormal morphology of QRS complexes appears prematurely without a preceding P′ waves. The compensatory pauses are complete. A sinus QRS complex is followed by a premature QRS complex.

ECG Interpretation

Sinus rhythm, bigeminal ventricular premature complex.

Premature beats may occur singularly and sporadically, or follow a specific pattern. "Bigeminy" and "trigeminy" are descriptors for a regular pattern. The premature beat may produce a bigeminy, a continuous pattern of a sinus beat followed by a premature beat, or a trigeminy, a continuous pattern of two sinus beats followed by a premature beat or a sinus beat followed by two premature beats. In this ECG, as in bigeminy, each sinus QRS complex is followed by a VPC (see Fig. 51-1).

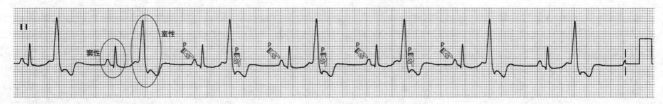

图51-1　室性期前收缩二联律

Fig. 51-1　Bigeminal ventricular premature complex

图例 52　室性期前收缩连发

Case 52　Couplet of Ventricular Premature Complexes

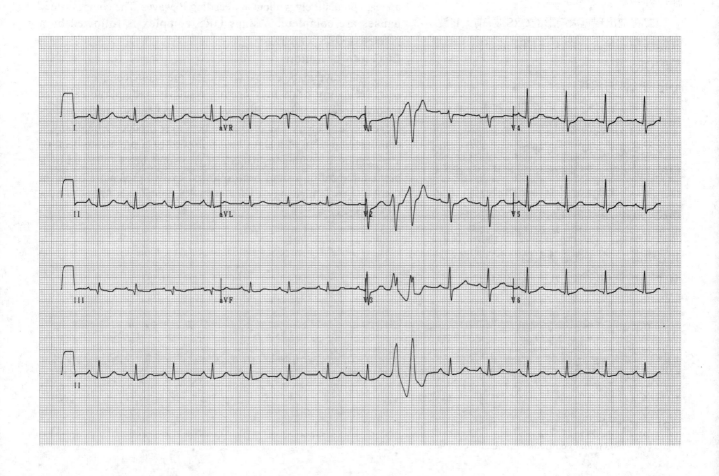

心电图特点

1. 心率: 88次/min; PR间期: 164 ms; QRS波时间: 88 ms; QT/QTc间期: 364/441 ms; QRS波电轴: 36°。

2. 成对提前出现宽大畸形的QRS波, 前无P'波。提前的QRS波形态相同。

心电图诊断与解析

诊断: 窦性心律; 室性期前收缩连发。

解析: 期前收缩可以单个发生, 也可连续重复发生, 如连发(连续两个)、三连发(连续三个)或连续更多期前收缩, 也称为短阵异位心动过速(详见图例54)。此心电图上有一对室性期前收缩, 称为室性期前收缩连发(见图52-1)。其QRS波形态相同, 表明起源相同。

ECG Characteristics

1. HR: 88 bpm; PR: 164 ms; QRS D: 88 ms; QT/QTc: 364/441 ms; QRS axis: 36°.

2. A pair of wide QRS complexes of abnormal morphology appears prematurely without a preceding P' wave. The morphologies of the premature QRS complexes are the same.

ECG Interpretation

Sinus rhythm, couplet of ventricular premature complexes.

Premature beats may occur isolated, or may also occur in a repetitive form: as couplet (two), triplet (three) or more in series, also defined as a short run of ectopic tachycardia (for details, see case 59). In this ECG, there is a pair of VPCs, which is a VPC couplet (see Fig. 52-1). The morphologies of the QRS complexes are the same, indicating that they have the same site of origin.

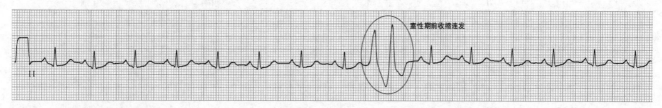

图52-1　室性期前收缩连发

Fig. 52-1　Ventricular premature complex's couplet

图例 53　多源性室性期前收缩连发

Case 53　Multifocal Ventricular Premature Complex's Couplet

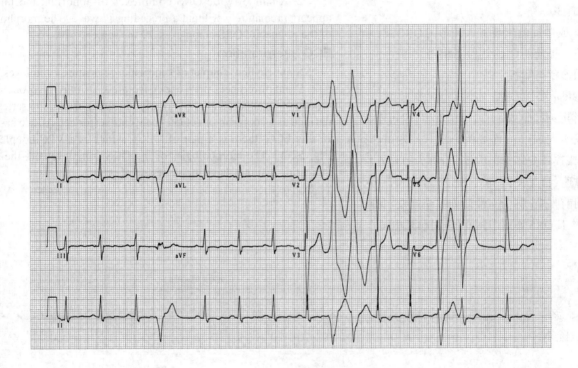

心电图特点

1. 心率：83次/min；PR间期：166 ms；QRS波时间：110 ms；QT/QTc间期：385/454 ms；QRS波电轴：40°。

2. 成对提前出现宽大畸形的QRS波，前

ECG Characteristics

1. HR: 83 bpm; PR: 166 ms; QRS D: 110 ms; QT/QTc: 385/454 ms; QRS axis: 40°.

2. Two pairs of wide and abnormal morphology QRS complexes appear prematurely without a preceding P′ waves. The morphologies of the premature QRS complexes are similar or different.

无P'波。提前的QRS波形态相同或不相同。

3. V1导联Ptf绝对值 > 0.04 mm · s。V5导联R波振幅 > 2.5 mV，$R_{V5}+S_{V1}$ > 3.5 mV，$R_{aVL}+S_{V3}$ > 2.8 mV。T波在Ⅱ、Ⅲ、aVF和V4 ~ V6导联低平。V6导联ST段压低 ≥ 0.05 mV。

心电图诊断与解析

诊断：窦性心律；室性期前收缩；多源性室性期前收缩连发；左心房肥大；左心室肥大；ST-T改变。

解析：此心电图上有两对室性期前收缩，QRS波形态前者相似，后者不同（见图53-1）。后者也可称为多源性或多形性室性期前收缩。QRS波形态不同表示室性期前收缩起源不同（多源性）或起源相同，但在心室中传导不同（多形性）。多源性和多形性的差别在于联律间期，通常多源性联律间期不等，多形性联律间期相等。

3. P-terminal force in lead V1 is > 0.04 mm·s. R wave in leads V5 is > 2.5 mV, $R_{V5} + S_{V1}$ > 3.5 mV, $R_{aVL} + S_{V3}$ > 2.8 mV. T waves are low and flat in leads Ⅱ, Ⅲ, aVF, and V4 ~ V6. ST segment depression in lead V6 is ≥ 0.05 mV.

ECG Interpretation

Sinus rhythm, ventricular premature complex, multifocal ventricular premature complex's couplet, left atrial enlargement, left ventricular hypertrophy, ST-T abnormalities.

In this ECG, there are two pairs of VPCs. The first pair has similar and the second has different morphologies of QRS complexes (see Fig. 53-1). The second pair is also called multifocal or multiform VPCs. The different morphologies of QRS complexes indicate that the VPCs have originated from different ectopic sites (multifocal) or from the same site but have had different conductions through the ventricles (multiform). The difference between the two situations is at the coupling interval. While the multiform VPCs usually have the same coupling intervals, multifocal VPCs tend to differ.

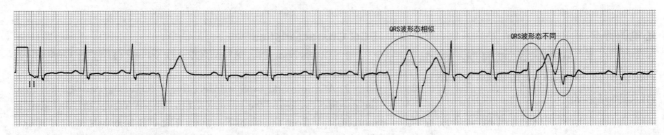

图53-1 多源性室性期前收缩连发

Fig. 53-1 Multifocal ventricular premature complex's couplet

图例54　短阵房性心动过速

Case 54　Short Run of Atrial Tachycardia

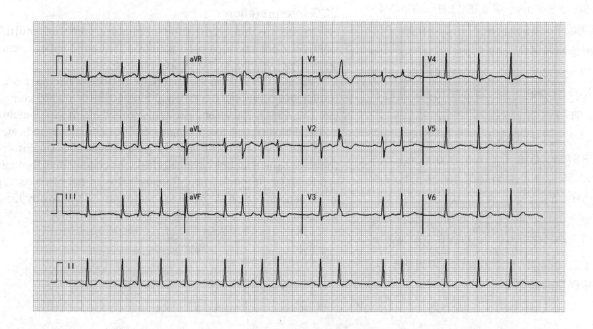

心电图特点

1. 心率：88次/min；PR间期：187 ms；QRS波时间：99 ms；QT/QTc间期：370/448 ms；QRS波电轴：68°。

2. 基本节律中提前出现单个或连续的P′波。P′波形态与窦性P波不同。P′R间期 > 120 ms。P′波后QRS波形态正常或宽大

ECG Characteristics

1. HR: 88 bpm; PR: 187 ms; QRS D: 99 ms; QT/QTc: 370/448 ms; QRS axis: 68°.

2. A single and three consecutive P′ waves appear earlier than the cardiac cycles of the basic rhythm. The P′ waves are different in morphology from the sinus P waves. The P′R intervals are > 120 ms. The P′ waves are followed by QRS complexes, normal or wide with abnormal morphology. The compensatory pauses are incomplete.

畸形。代偿间期不完全。

心电图诊断与解析

诊断：窦性心律；房性期前收缩伴心室内差异传导；短阵房性心动过速。

解析：三个或三个以上连续出现的快速异位心动称为异位心动过速。异位心动过速有两种类型。常见的类型是阵发性心动过速，突然发生和终止，发作时心率较快。不常见的类型是非阵发性心动过速，心率逐渐增加或减慢，而非突然发生和终止，发作时心率较慢。异位心动过速可以起源于心房，房室交界区或心室。房性心动过速起源于心房，通常心房率在100～250次/min，P′波形态与窦性P波不同。此心电图上房性心动过速由三个连续的P′波组成，称为短阵房性心动过速（见图54-1）。

ECG Interpretation

Sinus rhythm, atrial premature complex with aberrant intraventricular conduction, short run of atrial tachycardia.

Three or more consecutive ectopic beats are termed ectopic tachycardia. There are two types of ectopic tachycardia. The more common type is the paroxysmal tachycardia, with abrupt onset and termination and faster heart rate during the episode. The less common type is the non-paroxysmal tachycardia, gradual increase or decrease in heart rate instead of abrupt onset and termination, slower heart rate during the episode. Ectopic tachycardia may originate from the atria, A–V junction or the ventricles. Atrial tachycardia arises from an ectopic source in the atria and generally produces an atrial rate of 100 ~ 250 bpm. The P′ wave can be different in morphology from the sinus P wave depending on the ectopic site. In this ECG, the atrial tachycardia comprises three consecutive P′ waves, and it is called a short run of atrial tachycardia(see Fig. 54-1).

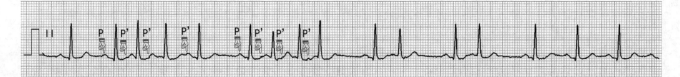

图54-1　短阵房性心动过速

Fig. 54-1　Short run of atrial tachycardia

图例55　阵发性房性心动过速

- -

Case 55　Paroxysmal Atrial Tachycardia

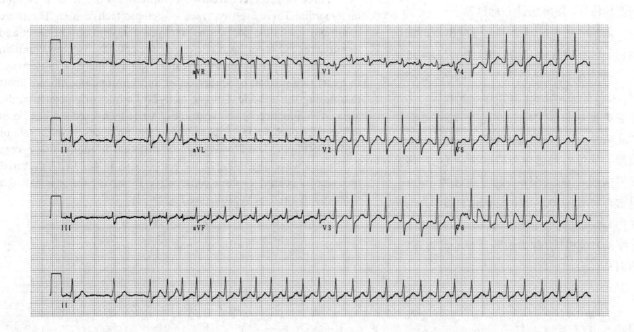

心电图特点

1. 心率：88次/min；PR间期：140 ms；QRS波时间：98 ms；QT/QTc间期：340/412 ms；QRS波电轴：20°。

2. 基本节律中出现快速的连续的P′波（187次/min）。P′波在Ⅱ导联直立，形态与窦性P波不同。P′R间期等于120 ms。P′波后

ECG Characteristics

1. HR: 88 bpm; PR: 140 ms; QRS D: 98 ms; QT/QTc: 340/412 ms; QRS axis: 20°.

2. Rapid and consecutive P′ waves appear earlier than the cardiac cycles of the basic rhythm (187 bpm). The P′ waves are upright in lead Ⅱ and different in morphology from the sinus P waves. The P′R intervals are equal to 120 ms. The P′ waves are followed by QRS complexes with normal morphology.

QRS波形态正常。

心电图诊断与解析

诊断：窦性心律；阵发性房性心动过速。

解析：起源于心房或交界区的阵发性心动过速统称为阵发性室上性心动过速。室上性心动过速应该被分为房性和交界性心动过速，鉴别诊断主要依赖P′波的形态。但是当心动过速心率太快时，P′波重叠在T波中，很难识别和鉴别诊断。在临床上，阵发性室上性心动过速被保留用于房性和交界性心动过速。此心电图上可见阵发性房性心动过速的三项特征。第一，可见心动过速突然发生，心房率高达187次/min。第二，P′波在Ⅱ导联直立，形态与窦性P波不同，V1导联也可见清晰的P′波。P′波在QRS波前，P′R间期等于120 ms。第三，心房律和心室律规则，1∶1传导（见图55-1）。

ECG Interpretation

Sinus rhythm, paroxysmal atrial tachycardia.

Any paroxysmal tachyarrhythmia arising from the atria or the A–V junction is a paroxysmal supraventricular tachycardia. Of course, supraventricular tachycardia should be divided into atrial and junctional tachycardia. The differential diagnosis is mainly dependant on the morphology of the P′ wave. But when the rate of tachycardia is so fast, the P′ wave merges into the T wave, leading to difficulty in recognizing the P′ wave and differentiating from each other. In clinical practice, however, the term paroxysmal supraventricular tachycardia is reserved for atrial and junctional tachycardias. In this ECG, there are three distinctive features of paroxysmal atrial tachycardia. First, tachycardia has an abrupt onset in atrial rate of 187 bpm. Second, the P′ waves are upright in lead Ⅱ and the morphology differs from that of sinus rhythm. The distinct P′ waves can also be seen in lead V1. The P′ waves precede the QRS complexes. The P′R intervals are equal to 120 ms. Third, the atrial and ventricular rhythms are regular with 1 : 1 ventricular response (1 : 1 conduction) (see Fig. 55-1).

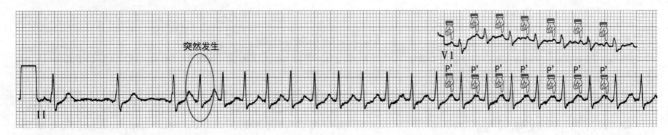

图55-1 阵发性房性心动过速

Fig. 55-1 Paroxysmal atrial tachycardia

图例56　阵发性房性心动过速（2∶1传导）

Case 56　Paroxysmal Atrial Tachycardia (2∶1 Conduction)

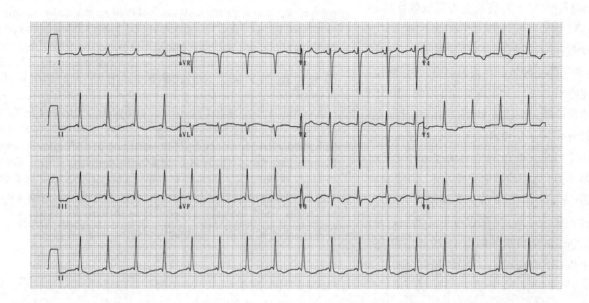

心电图特点

1. 心率：104次/min；PR间期：/；QRS波时间：96 ms；QT/QTc间期：350/460 ms；QRS波电轴：77°。

2. 连续的快速的P′波（208次/min）；P′P′间期规则，每两个P′波间隔一QRS波：一个P′波隐藏在T波中，另一个P′波紧靠QRS波。

3. QRS波形态正常。

ECG Characteristics

1. HR: 104 bpm; PR: /; QRS D: 96 ms; QT/QTc: 350/460 ms; QRS axis: 77°.

2. Rapid and consecutive P′ waves (208 bpm) occur; The P′P′ intervals are regular, every two P′ waves separated by one QRS complex: one P′ wave hidden in the T wave and the other close to the QRS complex.

3. The QRS complexes have normal morphology.

心电图诊断与解析

诊断：阵发性房性心动过速（2∶1传导）。

解析：此心电图上出现连续快速的P波，PP间期规则。如此快速的心房率（208次/min），应考虑诊断为房性心动过速。此心动速的特点是每两个P'波间隔一个QRS波，一个P'波隐藏在T波中，这是可能传导至心室的P'波，而另一个P'波紧靠QRS波，是不能传导至心室的（被阻断）P波，结果是房性心动过速呈2∶1传导（阻滞）（见图56-1）。按照规定，12导联心电图被分成三行四列来打印，前两列为肢体导联，后两列为胸前导联。每一片段心电图都是短阵的，根据心率不同，大约仅有1～3个心动，有时难以分析心律失常。为了有助分析，常在心电图记录纸的底部打印长的"节律条图"。通常是Ⅱ导联，或者是V1导联，都能清晰显示P或P'波（见图56-1）。

ECG Interpretation

Paroxysmal atrial tachycardia (2 : 1 conduction).

In this ECG, rapid and consecutive P' waves are present with regular P'P' interval. The atrial rate is so fast (208 bpm) that atrial tachycardia should highly be considered as diagnosis. In this tachycardia, every two P' waves are separated by one QRS complex. One P' wave is hidden in the T wave, which may be conducted to the ventricles. The other P' wave is close to the QRS complex, and may not be conducted (blocked). As a result, the atrial tachycardia is 2 : 1 conducted (or blocked) (see Fig. 56–1). By definition, a 12-lead ECG is often arranged in a grid of four columns by three rows, with the first two columns being the limb leads , and the last two columns being the precordial leads. Each of these segments is short, about one to three beats depending on the heart rate, making it difficult to analyze arrhythmias. To assist the analysis, a long "rhythm strip" is printed along the bottom of the ECG paper. It is usually with lead Ⅱ , sometimes with lead V1, and both of which show the P or P' wave well (see Fig. 56–1).

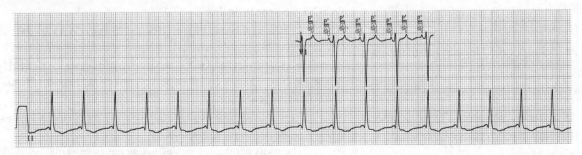

图56-1　房性心动过速2∶1传导

Fig. 56-1　Paroxysmal atrial tachycardia (2 : 1 conduction)

图例57 阵发性室上性心动过速

Case 57 Paroxysmal Supraventricular Tachycardia

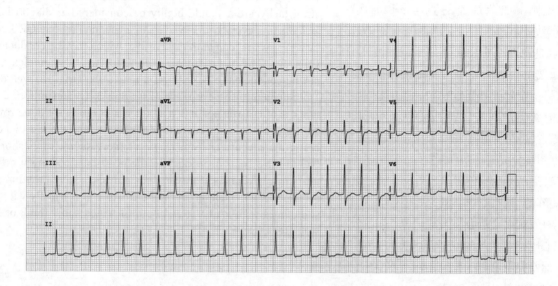

心电图特点

1. 心率：164次/min；PR间期：/；QRS波时间：75 ms；QT/QTc间期：280/462 ms；QRS波电轴：74°。

2. 规则的窄QRS波心动过速，心率 > 160次/min。Ⅱ、Ⅲ和aVF导联QRS波终末可见"S"波。

心电图诊断与解析

诊断：阵发性室上性心动过速（考虑阵

ECG Characteristics

1. HR: 164 bpm; PR: /; QRS D: 75 ms; QT/QTc: 280/462 ms; QRS axis: 74°.

2. Regular narrow QRS complex tachycardia with a rate > 160 bpm. The QRS complexes end with an "S" waves in leads Ⅱ, Ⅲ, and aVF.

ECG Interpretation

Paroxysmal supraventricular tachycardia (Consider paroxysmal A–V nodal reentrant tachycardia).

The most common types of junctional tachycardia are A–V nodal reentrant tachycardia (AVNRT) and atrioventricular reentrant tachycardia (AVRT). In AVNRT, there are two functionally and anatomically distinct

发性房室结折返性心动过速）。

解析：最常见的交界性心动过速是房室结折返性心动过速（AVNRT）和房室折返性心动过速（AVRT）。AVNRT是指房室结存在功能性双径路，一条径路相对快速但不应期长（快径路），另一条径路相对慢速但不应期短（慢径路）。正常时，来自心房的冲动经快径路传导激动心室。当一个特定冲动，如房性早搏，在快径路遇到不应期被阻断，经慢径路下传至心室。当冲动经慢径路向心室下传中，若快径路不应期已过，结果冲动在房室结内折返，经快径路上传再次进入心房，这样就形成AVNRT。在这折返环路中，慢径路用于前传，快径路用于逆传，称为"慢-快型"折返。在这类心动过速中，逆传心房的P′波可位于QRS波终末，在Ⅱ、Ⅲ和aVF导联倒置，形成假S波，在V1导联直立，形成假R波，RP′间期<P′R间期，RP′间期<70 ms。此心电图上，Ⅱ、Ⅲ和aVF导联QRS波终末可见"S"波（见图57-1），考虑"S"波为逆传P′，则RP′间期<P′R间期，RP′间期<70 ms，提示AVNRT。

pathways (dual A–V nodal pathway) in the A–V node. One pathway is relatively fast and has a long refractory period (fast pathway) and the other pathway is slow with a short refractory period (slow pathway). Normally an impulse from atria is conducted through the fast pathway to activate ventricles. If a particular impulse, such as an APC, occurs when the fast pathway is still refractory, the impulse will be blocked in the fast pathway and be conducted through the slow pathway to the ventricles. While the impulse conducts to the ventricles in the slow pathway, if the fast pathway recovers from its refractory period so that the impulse will turn around in the A–V node and reenter up through the fast pathway to the atria. Thus an AVNRT is initiated. In this reentry circuit, slow pathway is used for antegrade conduction and fast pathway is used for retrograde conduction, so called slow-fast reentry. In this type of tachycardia, atrial retrograde P′ wave may be seen in the last part of the QRS complex, inverted in leads Ⅱ, Ⅲ, and aVF to form a pseudo S wave, and upright in lead V1 to form a pseudo R wave, RP′ interval is < P′R interval and RP′ interval is < 70 ms. In this ECG, the QRS complexes end with "S" waves in leads Ⅱ, Ⅲ, and aVF (see Fig. 57-1). Consider that the "S" wave is the retrograde P′ wave, so RP′ intervals are < P′R interval and RP′ intervals are < 70 ms, suggesting AVNRT.

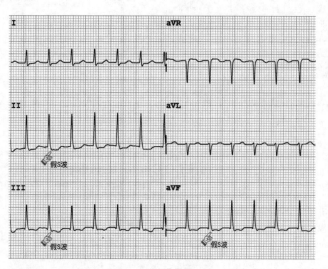

图57-1 阵发性房室结折返性心动过速

Fig. 57-1 Paroxysmal A–V nodal reentrant tachycardia

图例58 阵发性室上性心动过速

Case 58 Paroxysmal Supraventricular Tachycardia

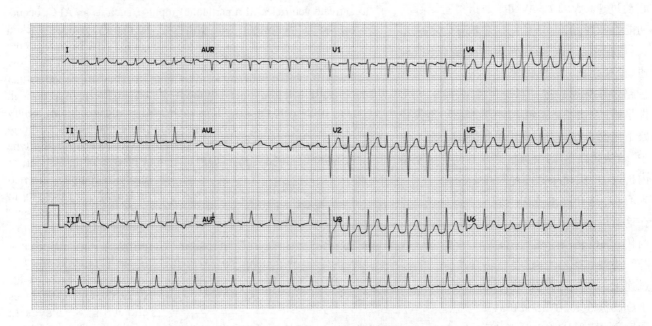

心电图特点

1. 心率：165次/min；PR间期：/；QRS波时间：92 ms；QT/QTc间期：270/445 ms；QRS波电轴：75°。

2. 规则的窄QRS波心动过速，心率＞160次/min。Ⅱ、Ⅲ和aVF导联可见倒置的P′波，RP′间期＜P′R间期，RP′间期＞70 ms。

ECG Characteristics

1. HR: 165 bpm; PR: /; QRS D: 92 ms; QT/QTc: 270/445 ms; QRS axis: 75°.

2. Regular narrow QRS complex tachycardia with a rate > 160 bpm. Inverted P′ waves are seen in leads Ⅱ, Ⅲ, and aVF, RP′ intervals are < P′R and RP′ intervals are > 70 ms.

ECG Interpretation

Paroxysmal supraventricular tachycardia (consider paroxysmal

心电图诊断与解析

诊断：阵发性室上性心动过速（考虑阵发性房室折返性心动过速）。

解析：心房和心室之间可能存在由旁道介入的解剖相连，由此发生 AVRT。旁道使得心房的冲动绕开房室结，提前激动心室，称为心室预激（详见图例94和95）。旁道相对快速但不应期长，房室结慢速但不应期短。旁道构成折返环路，可以形成窄 QRS 波或宽 QRS 波心动过速，取决于前传是经房室结还是经旁道。通常冲动在旁道中被阻断，经正常房室结下传至心室，然后冲动折返经旁道逆传至心房。由于前传是经房室结，形成窄 QRS 波心动过速，RP′间期<P′R 间期，通常 RP′间期 ≥ 70 ms。此心电图上，Ⅱ、Ⅲ 和 aVF 导联倒置的 P′波清晰可见，RP′间期<P′R 间期，RP′ > 70 ms，提示 AVRT（见图 58-1）。

A–V reentrant tachycardia).

Atria and ventricles may have an anatomically distinct A–V connection with circuits involving accessory pathway, resulting in AVRT. The accessory pathway allows the atrial impulse to bypass the A–V node to activate the ventricles prematurely, called ventricular preexcitation (for details, see case 94 and 95). The accessory pathway is relatively fast and has a long refractory period and the A–V node is slow and has a short refractory period. The accessory pathway allows the formation of a reentry circuit, which may give rise to either a narrow or a broad complex tachycardia, depending on whether the A–V node or the accessory pathway is used for antegrade conduction. Generally the impulse is blocked in the accessory pathway and conducted through the A–V node to the ventricles, and then the impulse reenters retrogradely via an accessory pathway to the atria, resulting in a narrow QRS complex tachycardia with RP′ interval < P′R interval. Generally, RP′ interval is ≥ 70 ms. In this ECG, inverted P′ waves are clearly seen in leads Ⅱ, Ⅲ and aVF, RP′ intervals are < P′R intervals and RP′ intervals are > 70 ms, suggesting AVRT (see Fig. 58-1).

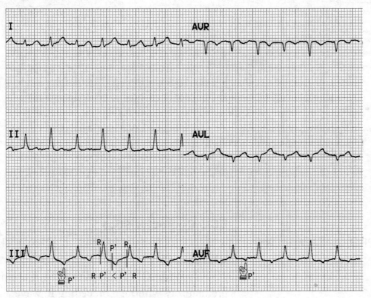

图 58-1　阵发性房室折返性心动过速

Fig. 58-1　Paroxysmal A–V reentrant tachycardia

图例 59   短阵室性心动过速

Case 59   Short Run of Ventricular Tachycardia

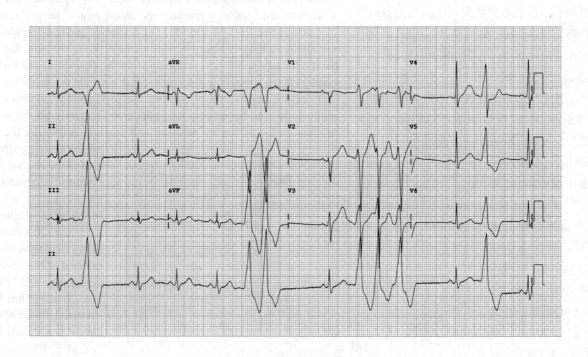

心电图特点

1. 心率: 71次/min; PR间期: 148 ms; QRS波时间: 110 ms; QT/QTc间期: 390/426 ms; QRS波电轴: 27°。

2. 提前出现宽大畸形的QRS波, 前无异位P波。

ECG Characteristics

1. HR: 71 bpm; PR: 148 ms; QRS D: 110 ms; QT/QTc: 390/426 ms; QRS axis: 27°.

2. Wide QRS complexes with abnormal morphology appear prematurely without a preceding P′ wave.

3. The premature QRS complexes are either single, in couplet, or in a short run.

3.提前的QRS波呈单个、连发和短阵发作。

心电图诊断与解析

诊断：窦性心律；室性期前收缩；室性期前收缩连发；短阵室性心动过速。

解析：如前所述（图例52），室性期前收缩可连续反复发生，三连发（连续三个）或连续更多，也称为短阵室性心动过速。在室性心动过速中，心室激动顺序发生改变，冲动不再沿着心室内传导系统传导，导致QRS波形态异常，时间延长，通常＞120 ms。此心电图上有两次单发室性期前收缩，一次室性期前收缩连发和一阵短阵室性心动过速。其QRS波形态相同，表明起源相同（见图59-1）。

ECG Interpretation

Sinus rhythm, ventricular premature complex, couplet of ventricular premature complexes, short run of ventricular tachycardia.

As mentioned before (case 52), VPCs may occur in a repetitive form as triplet (three) or more consecutive premature beats, also called a short run of ventricular tachycardia. In ventricular tachycardia the sequence of ventricular activation is altered, and the impulse no longer follows the normal intraventricular conduction pathway. As a result, the morphology of the QRS complex is abnormal, and the duration of the complex is prolonged, usually to 120 ms or longer. In this ECG, there are two isolated VPCs, one VPCs couplet, and one short run of ventricular tachycardia (see Fig. 59-1). The morphology of the QRS complexes is the same, indicating originated from the same site.

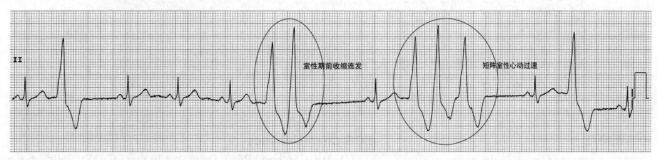

图59-1　室性期前收缩连发和短阵室性心动过速

Fig. 59-1　Couplet of ventricular premature complexes and short run of ventricular tachycardia

图例60 阵发性室性心动过速

Case 60 Paroxysmal Ventricular Tachycardia

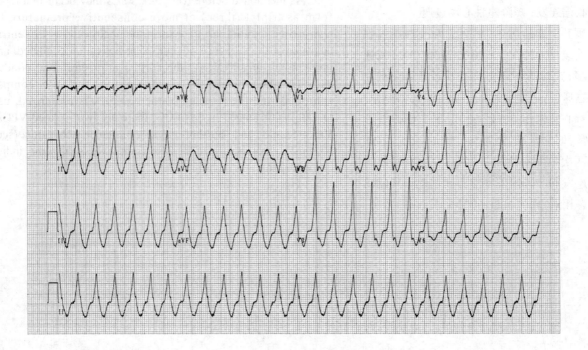

心电图特点

1. 心率：156次/min；PR间期：/；QRS波时间：170 ms；QT/QTc间期：350/564 ms；QRS波电轴：92°。

2. 出现连续的宽QRS波，频率＞130次/min。

3. 节律规则，QRS波形态相同。

ECG Characteristics

1. HR: 156 bpm; PR: /; QRS D: 170 ms; QT/QTc: 350/564 ms; QRS axis: 92°.

2. Consecutive wide QRS complexes with rate > 130 bpm.

3. Regular rhythm and consistent QRS complex morphology.

ECG Interpretation

Paroxysmal ventricular tachycardia.

心电图诊断与解析

诊断：阵发性室性心动过速。

解析：根据QRS波形态，心动过速可以被分为窄QRS波和宽QRS波。宽QRS波心动过速可以起源于心室，也可以起源于心室以上。在宽QRS波心动过速诊断上，最重要的是判断心动过速是否是心室起源，因为心室起源的心动过速预后不良。然而，用于诊断的规则相当复杂，而且不能适用于所有病例。经典的室性心动过速，QRS波时间≥120 ms，频率在130～200次/min之间，RR间期规则或偶尔不规则。一般而言，QRS波越宽，心室起源的可能性越大，尤其是波宽>160 ms。若有以往心电图资料，与宽QRS波心动过速比较，有助于诊断。室性心动过速可以终止，恢复至窦性心律。假如恢复为窦性心律，在窦性心律中若有室性期前收缩，窦性心动的QRS波和室性期前收缩的QRS波与宽QRS波心动过速比较，也有助于诊断。此心电图上，QRS波时间>160 ms，第一印象是室性心动过速。在随后的心电图记录中，心动过速突然终止，其QRS波形态与窦性心动的QRS波明显不同，而与室性期前收缩的QRS波相同（见图60-1)，室性心动过速进一步被肯定。

Tachycardia may be classified into narrow and broad complex based on the QRS complex. Broad QRS complex tachycardia may be ventricular or supraventricular in origin. The most important aspect of diagnosing broad QRS complex tachycardia is determining whether or not the tachycardia is ventricular, since ventricular tachycardia carries the worst prognosis. However, the criteria for a diagnosis of ventricular tachycardia are so complex that they are not satisfied in many cases. Classical ventricular tachycardia has QRS duration ≥ 120 ms and a rate ranging from 130 to 200 bpm. RR intervals are regular and occasionally irregular. As a general rule, the broader the QRS complex, the more likely the rhythm is to be ventricular in origin, especially if the complex duration is longer than 160 ms. If previous ECGs are available, comparing their morphologies with that of broad QRS complex tachycardia, it will be useful for making diagnosis. Ventricular tachycardia may end by reverting to sinus rhythm. If this occurs and if there is VPC during sinus rhythm, comparing the QRS complex morphologies of sinus beat and of VPC with that of broad QRS complex tachycardia, it will also be useful for making diagnosis. In this ECG, the QRS duration is > 160 ms, preliminarily suggesting ventricular tachycardia. Then, the tachycardia ends suddenly in the next ECG recording (see Fig. 60-1), with QRS complex morphology quite different in sinus rhythm and the same as VPCs. The diagnosis of ventricular tachycardia is thus further confirmed.

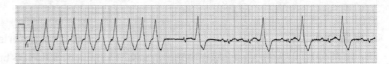

图 60-1 阵发性室性心动过速终止

Fig. 60-1 Paroxysmal ventricular tachycardia ends

图例61 阵发性室性心动过速

Case 61 Paroxysmal Ventricular Tachycardia

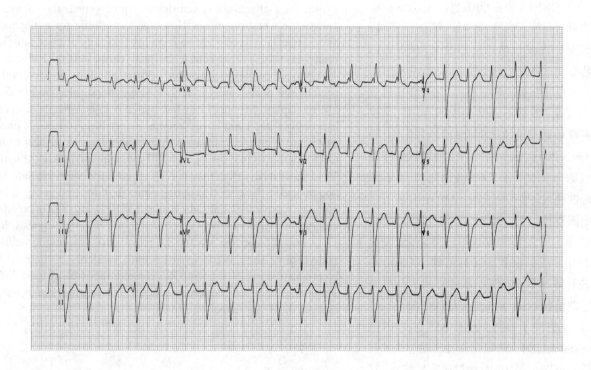

心电图特点

1. 心 率：123次/min；PR间 期：/；QRS波时间：142 ms；QT/QTc间期：374/535 ms；QRS波电轴：−87°。

2. 出现连续的宽QRS波，节律规则，QRS

ECG Characteristics

1. HR: 123 bpm; PR: /; QRS D: 142 ms; QT/QTc: 374/535 ms; QRS axis: −87°.

2. Consecutive wide QRS complexes appear in regular rhythm and consistent morphology.

3. The dissociated P waves are upright in lead Ⅱ.

波形态相同。

3. 与QRS波无关的P波在Ⅱ导联上直立。

心电图诊断与解析

诊断：阵发性室性心动过速。

解析：在室性心动过速中，窦房结继续激动心房，心房律和心室律各自独立。由于心房激动和心室激动各自独立，结果是房室分离，P波与QRS波无关。无关的P波在Ⅰ和Ⅱ导联中直立，通常心房率低于心室率。房室分离是心房独立激动的直接征象，只有当心动过速的心率<150次/min，才便于识别。心率过快，很难发现P波。因此，虽然房室分离征象对室性心动过速有诊断意义，但是缺乏房室分离的征象，并不能排除诊断。此心电图上，宽QRS波心动过速的频率为123次/min，很容易发现无关的P波，P波在Ⅱ导联中直立（见图61-1），室性心动过速的诊断可以被肯定。

ECG Interpretation

Paroxysmal ventricular tachycardia.

During ventricular tachycardia, the sinus node continues to activate the atria. Thus atrial and ventricular rhythms are independent of each other. This atrial activity is completely independent of ventricular activity, resulting in A–V dissociation, the P wave is dissociated from the QRS complex. The dissociated P wave is upright in leads Ⅰ and Ⅱ. The atrial rate is usually slower than the ventricular rate. A–V dissociation is direct evidence of independent atrial activity and is only easily recognized if the rate of tachycardia is < 150 bpm. Faster heart rates make it difficult to visualize dissociated P wave. Therefore, although evidence of A–V dissociation is diagnostic for ventricular tachycardia, a lack of it does not exclude the diagnosis. In this ECG, the rate of broad QRS complex tachycardia is 123 bpm. Dissociated P waves are easily to find and upright in lead Ⅱ (see Fig. 61-1). Ventricular tachycardia is then confirmed.

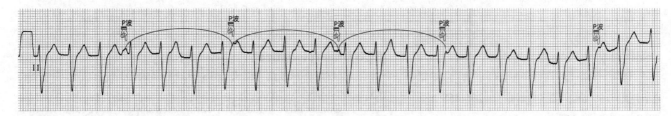

图61-1 室性心动过速与房室分离

Fig. 61-1 A–V dissociation in ventricular tachycardia

图例62 阵发性室性心动过速

Case 62 Paroxysmal Ventricular Tachycardia

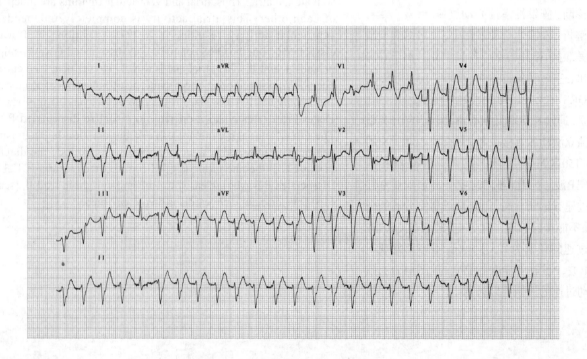

心电图特点

1. 心率：150次/min；PR间期：/；QRS波时间：139 ms；QT/QTc间期：296/468 ms；QRS波电轴：254°。

2. 出现连续的宽QRS波，节律规则，QRS波形态相同。

ECG Characteristics

1. HR: 150 bpm; PR: /; QRS D: 139 ms; QT/QTc: 296/468 ms; QRS axis: 254°.

2. Consecutive wide QRS complexes appear in regular rhythm and consistent morphologies.

3. One early narrow QRS complex appears.

4. The dissociated P waves are upright in lead II.

3. 可见一次提前的窄QRS波。

4. 与QRS波无关的P波在Ⅱ导联上直立。

心电图诊断与解析

诊断：阵发性室性心动过速。

解析：如前所述（图例61），在室性心动过速中，窦房结继续激动心房。偶尔，一个心房激动可能通过正常的传导系统激动心室，结果是出现一个提早的、窄QRS波的心动，这一心动称为夺获，是心房独立激动的间接征象。夺获不常见，常发生在有房室分离时。尽管出现夺获能肯定室性心动过速的诊断，但是未出现夺获并不能排除诊断。此心电图上第五个心动是提早的窄QRS波，是一次夺获，同样也可见房室分离（见图62-1），强烈提示宽QRS波心动过速起源于心室。

ECG Interpretation

Paroxysmal ventricular tachycardia.

As mentioned before (case 61), during ventricular tachycardia, the sinus node continues to activate the atria. Occasionally an atrial impulse may pass through the normal conduction system and activate the ventricles, resulting that the QRS complex occurs earlier than expected and is narrow. Such a beat is called capture beat and is indirect evidence of independent atrial activity. Capture beat is uncommon and often occurs when there is A–V dissociation. Although it confirms a diagnosis of ventricular tachycardia, its absence does not exclude the diagnosis. In this ECG, the 5th beat is an early narrow QRS complex (see Fig. 62–1), thus a capture beat. A–V dissociation can also be seen, strongly suggests a ventricular origin for the broad QRS complex tachycardia.

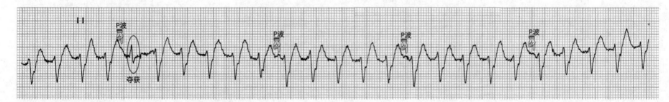

图62-1 室性心动过速与房室分离和夺获

Fig. 62–1 A–V dissociation and capture beat in ventricular tachycardia

图例63 非阵发性房性心动过速

Case 63 Non-paroxysmal Atrial Tachycardia

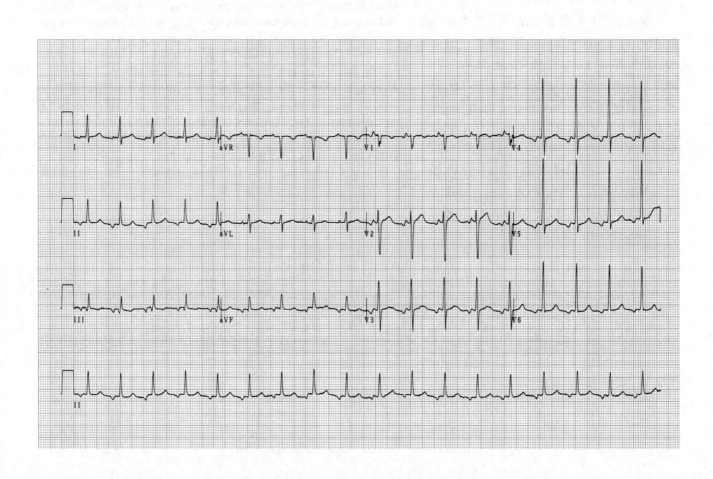

心电图特点

1. 心率：108 次/min；PR 间期：146 ms；QRS 波时间：76 ms；QT/QTc 间期：316/423 ms；QRS 波电轴：53°。

2. 快速的连续的 P′波，P′P′间期相等。P′波在 Ⅱ 导联上倒置，在 aVR 导联上直立。

3. P′R 间期 > 120 ms。

4. P′波后 QRS 波形态正常。

心电图诊断与解析

诊断：非阵发性房性心动过速。

解析：非阵发性心动过速是心动过速少见的类型。这类心动过速同样可以起源于心房、交界区和心室。非阵发性心动过速的发作通常是逐渐和缓慢的，非阵发性房性或交界性心动过速的频率为 70~130 次/min，非阵发性室性心动过速的频率为 60~100 次/min。此心电图上，心动过速的频率是 108 次/min，P′波在 Ⅱ 导联上倒置，在 aVR 导联上直立，P′R 间期 > 120 ms，因此这一心动过速可能起源于心房（见图 63-1）。

ECG Characteristics

1. HR: 108 bpm; PR: 146 ms; QRS D: 76 ms; QT/QTc: 316/423 ms; QRS axis: 53°.

2. Rapid and consecutive P′ waves appear with regular P′P′ interval. The P′ waves are inverted in lead Ⅱ and upright in lead aVR.

3. The P′R intervals are > 120 ms.

4. The P′ waves are followed by normal QRS complexes.

ECG Interpretation

Non-paroxysmal atrial tachycardia.

Non-paroxysmal tachycardia is a rare type of tachycardia, and also may originate from the atria, A–V junction or ventricles. The onset of non-paroxysmal tachycardia is usually gradual and slow. The heart rates range from 70 to 130 bpm for non-paroxymal atrial or junctional tachycardia, ranges from 60 to 100 bpm for non-paroxysmal ventricular tachycardia. In this ECG, the rate of tachycardia is 108 bpm, the P′ waves are inverted in lead Ⅱ and upright in lead aVR, the P′R intervals are > 120 ms, therefore this tachycardia might originate from the atria (see Fig. 63-1).

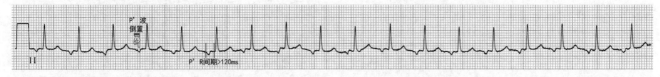

图 63-1 非阵发性房性心动过速

Fig. 63-1 Non-paroxysmal atrial tachycardia

图例64　非阵发性交界性心动过速

Case 64　Non-paroxysmal Junctional Tachycardia

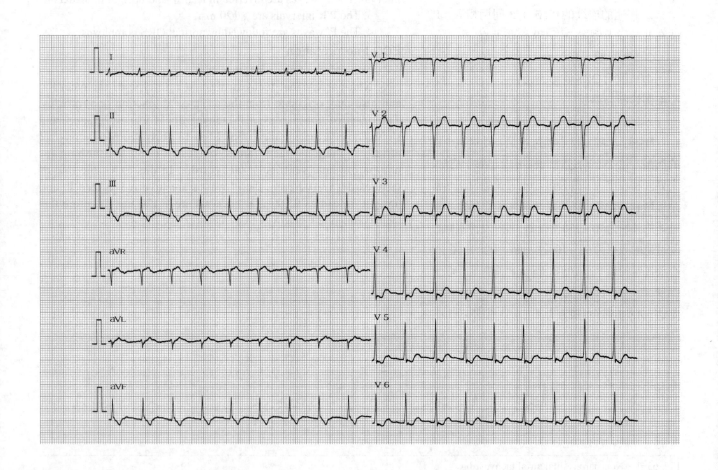

心电图特点

1. 心率：120次/min；PR间期：/；QRS波时间：78 ms；QT/QTc间期：320/423 ms；QRS波电轴：79°。

2. 窄QRS波心动过速，P′P′间期规则，心率为120次/min。P′波在Ⅱ导联上倒置，在aVR导联上直立。P′波在QRS波后，RP′间期<200 ms。

心电图诊断与解析

诊断：非阵发性交界性心动过速。

解析：此心电图上，心动过速的心率为120次/min，P′波在Ⅱ导联上倒置，在aVR导联上直立，P′波在QRS波后，RP′<200 ms，提示这一心动过速起源于房室交界区（见图64-1）。

ECG Characteristics

1. HR: 120 bpm; PR: /; QRS D: 78 ms; QT/QTc: 320/423 ms; QRS axis: 79°.

2. Narrow QRS complex tachycardia appears with a rate of 120 bpm and regular P′P′ interval. The P′ waves are inverted in lead Ⅱ and upright in lead aVR. The P′ waves are located after the QRS complexes and the RP′ intervals are < 200 ms.

ECG Interpretation

Non-paroxysmal junctional tachycardia.

In this ECG, the rate of tachycardia is 120 bpm, the P′ wave is inverted in lead Ⅱ and upright in lead aVR, and the P′ wave is located after the QRS complex with the RP′ interval < 200 ms, suggesting that this tachycardia originate from the A–V junction (see Fig. 64–1).

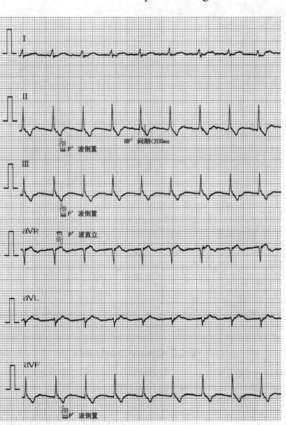

图64-1　非阵发性交界性心动过速

Fig. 64-1　Non-paroxysmal junctional tachycardia

图例65　非阵发性室性心动过速

Case 65　Non-paroxysmal Ventricular Tachycardia

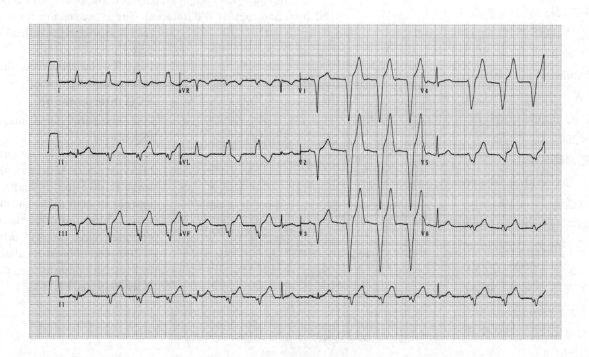

心电图特点

1. 心率: 96次/min; PR间期: 200 ms; QRS波时间: 136 ms; QT/QTc间期: 394/497 ms; QRS波电轴: −55°。

2. 出现连续的宽QRS波, 频率<100次/min。

3. 可见两次提前的窄QRS波。

ECG Characteristics

1. HR: 96 bpm; PR: 200 ms; QRS D: 136 ms; QT/QTc: 394/497 ms; QRS axis: −55°.

2. Consecutive wide QRS complexes, rate is < 100 bpm.

3. Two early narrow QRS complexes appear.

4. Three QRS complexes with morphology intermediate between narrow and broad QRS complexes appear.

4. 可见三次QRS波形态介于窄QRS波和宽QRS波之间。

心电图诊断与解析

诊断：窦性心律；非阵发性室性心动过速。

解析：此心电图宽QRS波心动过速有两项特征：夺获波和融合波。两者均是心房独立激动的间接征象。夺获前面已经解释过（图例62）。融合波是当窦性激动经房室结和希-浦氏系统向心室传导时，与心室起源的激动融合所形成的波。由于激动心室的冲动部分来自希-浦氏系统，部分来自心室，因此形成QRS波形态介于正常QRS波（窄）和心动过速的QRS波（宽）之间（见图65-1）。融合波不常见，易发生在频率缓慢的室性心动过速中。融合波支持室性心动过速的诊断。此心电图上可见两次夺获波和三次融合波，室性心动过速的频率<100次/min，属于非阵发性室性心动过速。

ECG Interpretation

Sinus rhythm, non-paroxysmal ventricular tachycardia.

In this ECG, two distinctive features of this broad tachycardia are capture beat and fusion beat, both indirect evidences of independent atrial activity. Capture beat is already mentioned before (case 62). A fusion beat occurs when a sinus impulse conducts to the ventricles via the A–V node and His-Purkinje system and fuses with an impulse arising in the ventricle. As the ventricles are activated partly by the impulse conducted through the His-Purkinje system and partly by the impulse arising in the ventricle, the resulting QRS complex has morphology intermediately between a normal beat (narrow) and a tachycardia beat (broad) (see Fig. 65-1). Fusion beat is uncommon and is likely to occur during slow rate ventricular tachycardia. Fusion beat supports a diagnosis of ventricular tachycardia. In this ECG, there are two capture beats and three fusion beats, the rate of ventricular tachycardia is < 100 bmp, belonging to non-paroxysmal ventricular tachycardia.

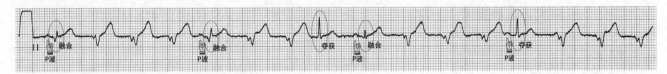

图 65-1 非阵发性室性心动过速中的夺获和融合

Fig. 65-1 Capture beat and fusion beat in non-paroxysmal ventricular tachycardia

图例66　心房扑动（2:1传导）

Case 66　Atrial Flutter (2:1 Block)

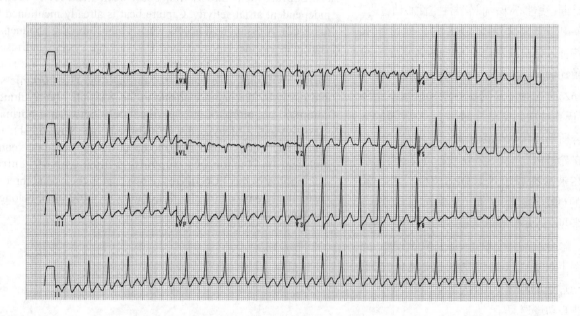

心电图特点

1. 心率：150次/min；PR间期：/；QRS波时间：80 ms；QT/QTc间期：256/404 ms；QRS波电轴：74°。

2. P波消失，心房波由快速规则的扑动波（F波）组成。F波呈锯齿样，在下壁导联和V1导联明显。

3. 心房率300次/min，心室率150次/min。

ECG Characteristics

1. HR: 150 bpm; PR: /; QRS D: 80 ms; QT/QTc: 256/404 ms; QRS axis: 74°.

2. The P waves are absent; the atrial deflections consist of rapid regular flutter (F) waves. The F waves appear saw-toothed and are best seen in the inferior leads and in lead V1.

3. The rate of atrial rhythm is 300 bpm and the ventricular rate is 150 bpm. The ventricular rhythm is regular. The QRS complexes have normal morphology.

心室律规则。QRS波形态正常。

心电图诊断与解析

诊断：心房扑动（2∶1传导）。

解析：心房扑动是一种快速的心房律（250～350次/min），P波消失，心房波由快速规则的扑动波（F）组成。起伏的F波之间没有等电位基线，在一些导联上呈锯齿样，尤其在下壁导联和V1导联。心室率取决于经房室结的传导。典型呈2∶1或4∶1传导，因此当心房率为300次/min时，心室率为150次/min或75次/min。心房扑动可以呈阵发性、持续性和永久性。尽管如此，心房扑动常是"一过性"的心律失常，常恢复窦性心律或转成心房颤动。此心电图上心房率是300次/min，心室率是150次/min（见图66-1），诊断为心房扑动（2∶1传导）。规则的心动过速，呈现这一频率（150次/min），应立即考虑诊断心房扑动。

ECG Interpretation

Atrial flutter (2∶1 block).

Atrial flutter is a fast atrial rhythm (250~350 bpm). The P waves become absent and the atrial deflections consist of rapid regular flutter (F) waves. The undulation F waves do not have an isoelectric baseline between them and give rise to a saw-tooth appearance in some leads, especially the inferior leads and lead V1. The ventricular rate depends on conduction through the A-V node. Typically 2∶1 or 4∶1 block (atrial rate to ventricular rate) occurs, giving a ventricular rate of 150 or 75 bpm when the atrial rate is 300 bpm. Atrial flutter may have paroxysmal, persistent and permanent forms. However, atrial flutter is a more "transient arrhythmia" that frequently changes to sinus rhythm or atrial fibrillation. In this ECG, the rate of atrial rhythm is 300 bpm and the ventricular rate is 150 bpm (see Fig. 66-1), so the diagnosis is atrial flutter (2∶1 block). Finding of a regular tachycardia with this rate (150 bpm) should prompt the diagnosis of atrial flutter.

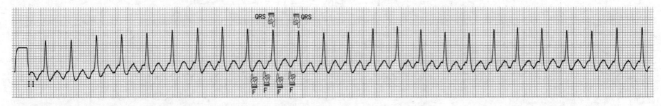

图66-1　心房扑动（2比1传导）

Fig. 66-1　Atrial flutter (2∶1 block)

图例67　心房扑动（4：1传导）

Case 67　Atrial Flutter (4:1 Block)

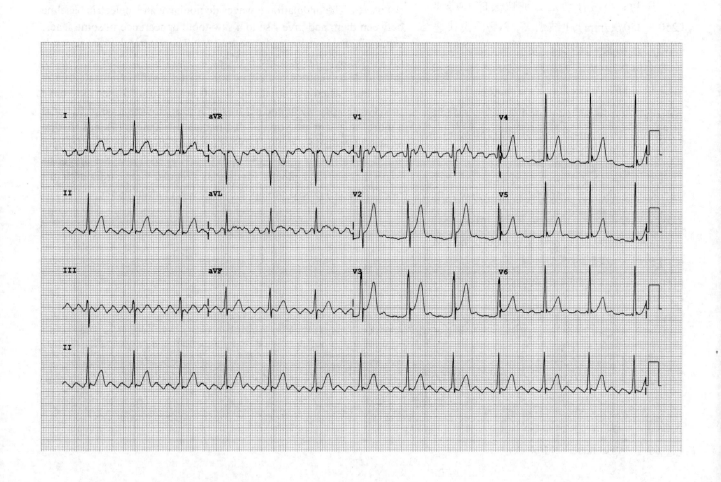

心电图特点

1. 心率：77次/min；PR间期：/；QRS波时间：100 ms；QT/QTc间期：340/385 ms；QRS波电轴：41°。

2. P波消失，心房波由快速规则的F组成。F波呈锯齿样，在下壁导联和V1导联明显。

3. 心房率308次/min，心室率77次/min。心室律规则。QRS波形态正常。

心电图诊断与解析

诊断：心房扑动（4∶1传导）。

解析：在心房扑动中，心室的频率和节律取决于房室传导的比例。假如房室传导比例是恒定的，则心室律是规则的。此心电图上心房扑动呈恒定的4∶1传导，心房率是308次/min，心室率是77次/min，心室律规则（见图67-1）。4∶1传导比例也是常见的，而3∶1和1∶1传导比例不常见。在4∶1传导比例时，F波清晰可见。

ECG Characteristics

1. HR: 77 bpm; PR: /; QRS D: 100 ms; QT/QTc: 340/385 ms; QRS axis: 41°.

2. The P waves are absent; the atrial deflections consist of rapid regular F waves. The F waves appear saw-toothed and are best seen in the inferior leads and in lead V1.

3. The rate of atrial rhythm is 308 bpm and the ventricular rate is 77 bpm. The ventricular rhythm is regular. The QRS complexes have normal morphology.

ECG Interpretation

Atrial flutter (4∶1 block).

In atrial flutter, the ventricular rate and regularity depend on the A–V conduction ratio. If the conduction ratio is constant, then the ventricular rhythm will be regular. In this ECG, the atrial flutter has a constant 4∶1 conduction ratio, the rate of atrial rhythm is 308 bpm and the ventricular rate is 77 bpm, and the ventricular rhythm is regular (see Fig. 67-1). 4∶1 conduction ratio is also common but 3∶1 and 1∶1 conduction ratio is uncommon. In 4∶1 conduction ratio the F waves become apparent.

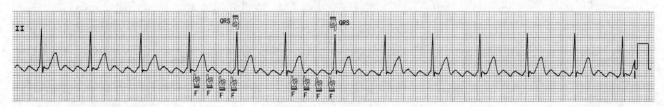

图67-1　心房扑动（4∶1传导）

Fig. 67-1　Atrial flutter (4∶1 block)

图例68 心房扑动(不等比传导)

Case 68　Atrial Flutter (Ventricular Response Irregular)

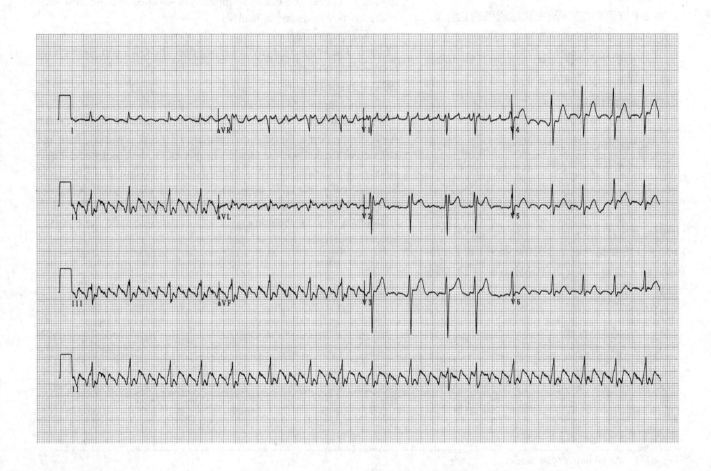

心电图特点

1. 心 率：102次/min；PR间期：/；QRS波时间：110 ms；QT/QTc间期：328/427 ms；QRS波电轴：63°。

2. P波消失，心房波由快速规则的F波组成。F波呈锯齿样，在下壁导联和V1导联明显。

3. 心室律不规则。

4. QRS波形态正常。

心电图诊断与解析

诊断：心房扑动（不等比传导）。

解析：有时心房扑动的房室传导比例是变化的，结果是心室律不规则。此心电图上心房扑动呈3∶1或4∶1传导，RR间期不等，结果是心室律不规则（见图68-1）。

ECG Characteristics

1. HR: 102 bpm; PR: /; QRS D: 110 ms; QT/QTc: 328/427 ms; QRS axis: 63°.

2. The P waves are absent; the atrial deflections consist of rapid regular F waves. The F waves appear saw-toothed and are best seen in the inferior leads and in lead V1.

3. The ventricular rhythm is irregular.

4. The QRS complexes have normal morphology.

ECG Interpretation

Atrial flutter (ventricular response irregular).

Sometimes, the A–V conduction ratio in atrial flutter is variable, and thus the ventricular rhythm is irregular. In this ECG, the atrial flutter has a conduction ratio changing between 3∶1 and 4∶1, the RR intervals are different, thus the ventricular rhythm is irregular (see Fig. 68-1).

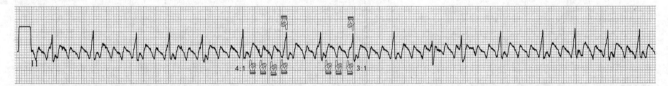

图68-1 心房扑动（不等比传导）

Fig. 68-1 Atrial flutter (ventricular response irregular)

图例69　阵发性心房扑动

Case 69　Paroxysmal Atrial Flutter

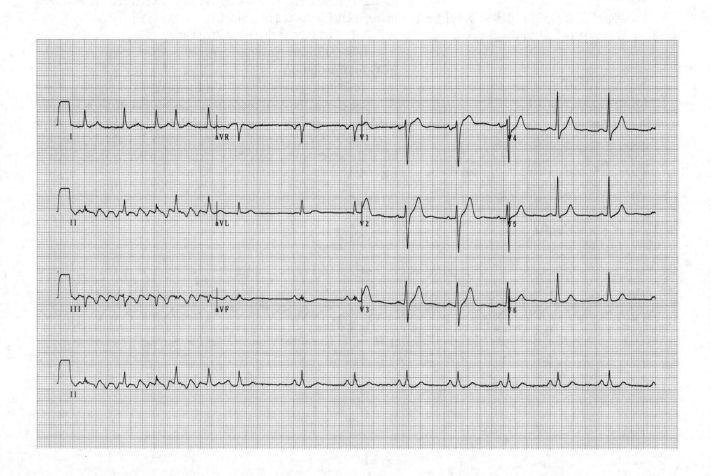

心电图特点

1. 心率: 68次/min; PR间期: 144 ms, QRS波时间: 94 ms; QT/QTc间期: 358/412 ms; QRS波电轴: 18°。

2. 阵发性心房扑动突然终止, 恢复至窦性心律。

心电图诊断与解析

诊断: 窦性心律; 阵发性心房扑动。

解析: 如前所述(图例66), 心房扑动通常是一种"一过性"的心律失常。此心电图上, 心房扑动突然终止, 恢复为窦性心律(见图69-1)。这就是阵发性心房扑动。

ECG Characteristics

1. HR: 68 bpm; PR: 144 ms; QRS D: 94 ms; QT/QTc: 358/412 ms; QRS axis: 18°.

2. Paroxysmal atrial flutter stops abruptly and converts to sinus rhythm.

ECG Interpretation

Sinus rhythm, paroxysmal atrial flutter.

As mentioned before (case 66), usually atrial flutter is a more transient arrhythmia. In this ECG, atrial flutter stops abruptly and converts to sinus rhythm (see Fig. 69-1). This is paroxysmal atrial flutter.

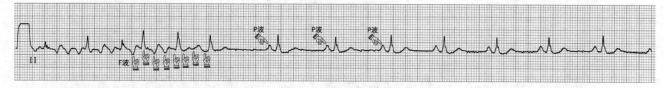

图69-1 阵发性心房扑动终止和窦性心律恢复

Fig. 69-1 Paroxysmal atrial flutter ends and converts to sinus rhythm

图例 70 心房颤动

Case 70 Atrial Fibrillation

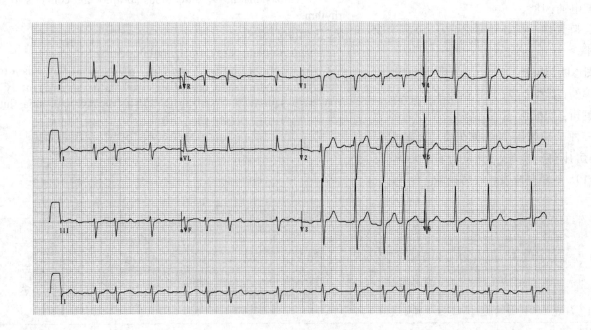

心电图特点

1. 心率：94次/min；PR间期：/；QRS波时间：110 ms；QT/QTc间期：370/462 ms；QRS波电轴：−42°。

2. P波消失，代之以小的振颤的颤动波（f波）。f波快速而且不规则。心室律绝对不规则。QRS波形态正常。电轴位于−30°以外。

ECG Characteristics

1. HR: 94 bpm; PR: /; QRS D: 110 ms; QT/QTc: 370/462 ms; QRS axis: −42°.

2. The P waves are absent, replaced by small and oscillating fibrillation (f) waves. The f waves are fast and irregular.

3. The ventricular rhythm is completely irregular.

4. The QRS complexes have normal morphology.

5. The axis lies beyond −30°.

心电图诊断与解析

诊断：心房颤动；电轴左偏。

解析：心房颤动是最常见的持续性心律失常。在心电图上可见P波被颤动波（f波）所取代。f波是小的振颤的波，快速（350～600次/min）而不规则。此类心房冲动向心室的传导是变化莫测的，只有少数冲动能经房室结传导产生不规则的心室反应。心室率取决于房室传导的程度。心室率通常是快速的（130～160次/min），而且节律绝对不规则。P波消失、f波和心室律不规则是心房颤动的特征。QRS波形态正常，若存在心室内差异传导、束支阻滞和心室预激，QRS波形态异常。此心电图上，P波消失、f波和不规则的心室反应，都指示心房颤动（见图70-1）。

ECG Interpretation

Atrial fibrillation, left axis deviation.

Atrial fibrillation is the most common sustained arrhythmia. It is seen on ECG as the fibrillation ("f") wave instead of the P waves. The "f" wave is small and oscillating, and also fast (350 ~ 600 bpm) and irregular. Conduction of such atrial impulses to the ventricles is variable and unpredictable. Only a few of the impulses transmit through the A-V node to produce an irregular ventricular response. The ventricular rate depends on the degree of A-V conduction. The rate is usually fast (130 ~ 160 bpm) with completely irregular rhythm. Combination of absent P waves, small f waves, and irregular ventricular complexes is characteristic of atrial fibrillation. The morphology of QRS complex is normal or abnormal if with aberrant conduction, bundle branch block or ventricular preexcitation. In this ECG, absent P waves, small f wave, and irregular ventricular response are all indicators of atrial fibrillation (see Fig. 70-1).

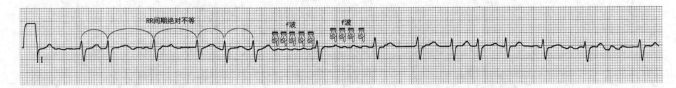

图70-1　心房颤动

Fig. 70-1　Atrial fibrillation

图例71　心房颤动伴快速心室率

Case 71　Atrial Fibrillation with Fast Ventricular Rate

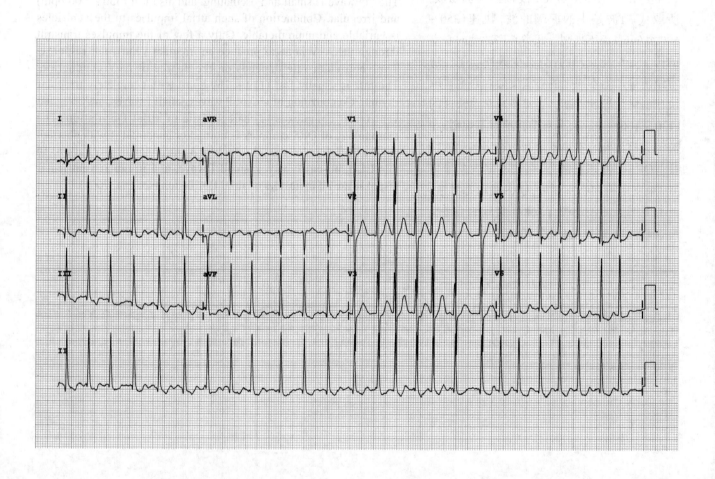

心电图特点

1. 心率：162次/min；PR间期：/；QRS波时间：79 ms；QT/QTc间期：292/479 ms；QRS波电轴：81°。

2. P波消失，代之以f波。颤动波快速而且不规则。心室率快速而且节律绝对不规则。QRS波形态正常。

心电图诊断与解析

诊断：心房颤动伴快速心室率。

解析：在心房颤动中，心室律绝对不规则，心室率不等，可以是快速的（心率＞100次/min）、中等的（60～100次/min）和缓慢的（＜60次/min）。此心电图上，心室率极快，节律不规则，因此心电图诊断为心房颤动伴快速心室率（见图71-1）。有时快室率心房颤动可能难以与其他类型的心动过速相鉴别。然而，RR间期仍可能不规则，越不规则，越可能是心房颤动。用分规测定RR间期，通常可以确定诊断。

ECG Characteristics

1. HR: 162 bpm; PR: /; QRS D: 79 ms; QT/QTc: 292/479 ms; QRS axis: 81°.

2. The P waves are absent, replaced by small f waves. The f waves are fast and irregular. The ventricular rate is fast and the rhythm is completely irregular. The QRS complexes have normal morphology.

ECG Interpretation

Atrial fibrillation with fast ventricular rate.

In atrial fibrillation, ventricular response is completely irregular and the rate is disparate, may be fast (HR > 100 bpm), moderate (HR=60 ~ 100 bpm) or slow (HR < 60 bpm). In this ECG, the ventricular rate is fast, the rhythm is completely irregular; therefore the ECG interpretation is atrial fibrillation with fast ventricular rate (see Fig. 71-1). Sometimes fast rate atrial fibrillation may be difficult to distinguish from other tachycardias. However, the RR interval remains irregular, the more irregular it is the more possible that is atrial fibrillation. Measuring RR intervals with caliper usually confirms the diagnosis.

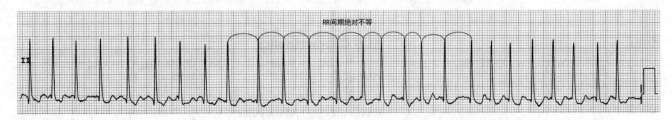

图71-1 心房颤动伴快速心室率

Fig. 71-1 Atrial fibrillation with fast ventricular rate

图例72　心房颤动伴长间期

Case 72　Atrial Fibrillation with Long Pause

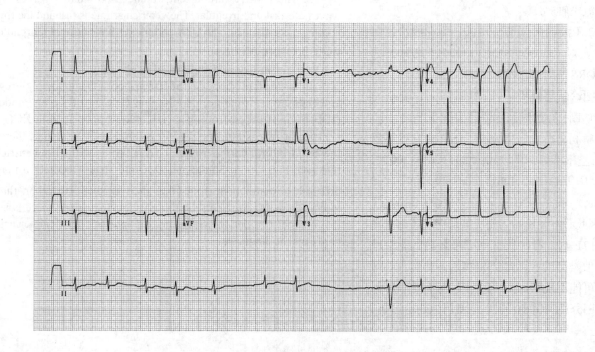

心电图特点

1. 心　率：76次/min；PR间　期：/；QRS波时间：88 ms；QT/QTc间期：352/396 ms；QRS波电轴：−29°。

2. P波消失，代之以f波。f波快速而且不规则。

ECG Characteristics

1. HR: 76 bpm; PR: /; QRS D: 88 ms; QT/QTc: 352/396 ms; QRS axis: −29°.

2. The P waves are absent, replaced by small f waves. The f waves are fast and irregular.

3. The ventricular rhythm is completely irregular and has a long pause.

4. The QRS complexes are normal except one beat after long pause.

3. 心室律绝对不规则,并可见一长间期。

4. QRS波形态正常。长间期后的QRS波形态异常。

心电图诊断与解析

诊断:心房颤动伴长间期;室性逸搏。

解析:在心房颤动中,由于f波不规则和f波存在不同程度的隐匿传导,心室率绝对不等。所谓隐匿传导是指f波未能通过房室交界区,但是仍能产生不应期,影响后续f波的传导。缓慢心室率或长间期提示高度房室阻滞,可能是由于房室结病变、药物作用或房室隐匿传导。此心电图上,可见一长间期,并在长间期后见一宽QRS波(见图72-1),提示心房颤动可能存在一定程度的房室传导阻滞。这一宽QRS波是室性逸搏,逸搏或逸搏心律(三次或更多心动)是一种被动机制形成的心律失常(详见图例79)。

ECG Interpretation

Atrial fibrillation with long pause, ventricular escape beat.

In atrial fibrillation, the ventricular rate is completely irregular due to the irregular f waves and the different degrees of concealed conduction of the f waves. The A-V concealed conduction occurs when the f wave does not cross the A-V junction completely, but still causes a refractory period, which has an effect on the conduction of successive f waves. Slow ventricular rate or a long pause suggests a high degree of A-V block, which may be caused by A-V node disease, medication effect or A-V concealed conduction. In this ECG, a long pause and a wide QRS complex at the end of pause (see Fig. 72-1) suggest this atrial fibrillation may have some degrees of A-V block. This wide QRS complex is a ventricular escape beat. The escape beat or rhythm (3 or more beats) is an arrhythmia due to passive mechanism (for details, see case 79).

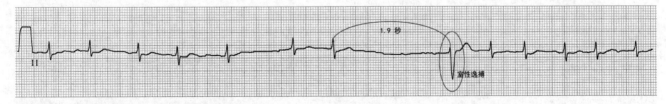

图72-1 心房颤动伴长间期和室性逸搏

Fig. 72-1 Atrial fibrillation with long pause and Ventricular escape beat

图例73 心房颤动伴三度房室传导阻滞

Case 73   Atrial Fibrillation with Third Degree A-V Block

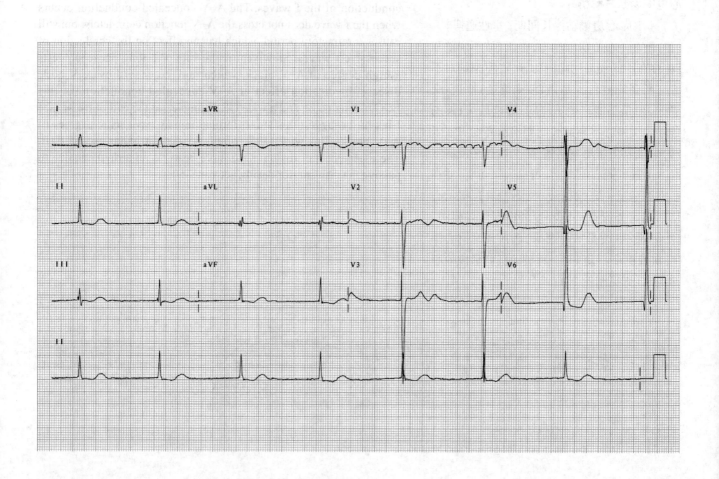

心电图特点

1. 心率：44次/min；PR间期：/；QRS波时间：95 ms；QT/QTc间期：540/462 ms；QRS波电轴：50°。

2. P波消失，代之以f波。f波快速而且不规则。心室律规则。QRS波形态正常。

心电图诊断与解析

诊断：心房颤动伴三度房室传导阻滞；交界性逸搏。

解析：心房颤动中心室率相等和缓慢，通常提示完全性（三度）房室传导阻滞和存在逸搏心律。若是交界性逸搏心律，QRS波形态正常（窄的），若是室性逸搏心律，QRS波形态异常（宽的）（见图例87）。此心电图上，心室率缓慢，节律规则，逸搏心律的QRS波形态正常，心电图诊断为心房颤动伴三度房室传导阻滞和交界性逸搏心律（见图73-1）。

ECG Characteristics

1. HR: 44 bpm; PR: /; QRS D: 95 ms; QT/QTc: 540/462 ms; QRS axis: 50°.

2. The P waves are absent, replaced by small f waves. The f waves are fast and irregular. The ventricular rhythm is regular. The QRS complexes have normal morphology.

ECG Interpretation

Atrial fibrillation with third degree A–V block, A–V junctional escape rhythm.

In atrial fibrillation, a regular and slow ventricular rhythm usually indicates complete (third degree) A–V block and presence of escape rhythm. QRS complexes are normal (narrow) for A–V junctional escape rhythm and abnormal (broad) for ventricular escape rhythm (see case 87). In this ECG, the ventricular rate is slow and the rhythm is regular, the QRS complexes in the escape rhythm are normal, and therefore the ECG interpretation is atrial fibrillation with third degree A–V block and A–V junctional escape rhythm (see Fig. 73–1).

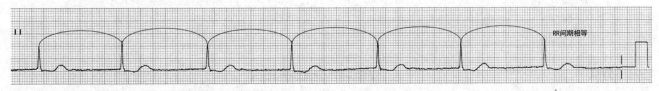

图73-1 心房颤动伴三度房室传导阻滞和交界性逸搏心律

Fig. 73-1 Atrial fibrillation with third degree A–V block and A–V junctional escape rhythm

图例74 阵发性心房颤动

Case 74 Paroxysmal Atrial Fibrillation

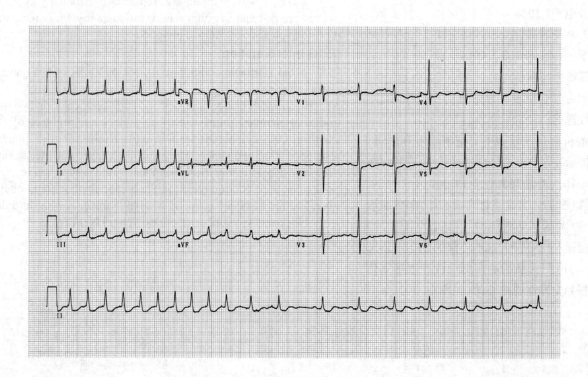

心电图特点

1. 心率: 83次/min; PR间期: 180 ms; QRS波时间: 82 ms; QT/QTc间期: 400/470 ms; QRS波电轴: 48°。

2. 心房颤动突然终止, 恢复至窦性心律。

ECG Characteristics

1. HR: 83 bpm; PR: 180 ms; QRS D: 82 ms; QT/QTc: 400/470 ms; QRS axis: 48°.

2. Arial fibrillation stops abruptly and converts to sinus rhythm.

3. ST segments depression in leads Ⅰ, Ⅱ, Ⅲ and aVF, V2 ~ V6 is > 0.05 mV. T waves are low and flat in leads V2 and V3.

3. Ⅰ、Ⅱ、Ⅲ、aVF和V2～V6导联ST段压低 > 0.05 mV。T波在V2和V3导联低平。

心电图诊断与解析

诊断：阵发性心房颤动；ST-T改变。

解析：心房颤动可以是阵发性、持续性或永久性。阵发性心房颤动突然发生，然后自行终止或治疗后终止，这类心房颤动可以持续数秒、数分、数小时或数天，但通常小于48 h。假如阵发性心房颤动持续大于48 h，很少能自行终止，但治疗后仍可能终止。持续性心房颤动是指心房颤动持续大于7天，这类心房颤动，治疗后仍可能终止，但也可能不能终止。永久性心房颤动，治疗后不能再恢复窦性心律。阵发性心房颤动和持续性心房颤动可逐步频发，最终成为永久性心房颤动。此心电图上，心房颤动突然终止，恢复为窦性心律（见图74-1），为阵发性心房颤动。

ECG Interpretation

Paroxysmal atrial fibrillation, ST-T abnormalities.

Atrial fibrillation may be paroxysmal, persistent, or permanent. Paroxysmal atrial fibrillation begins suddenly and then stops on its own or after treatment. This type of atrial fibrillation may last for seconds, minutes, hours, or days, but usually less than 48 hours. If paroxysmal atrial fibrillation continues more than 48 hours, it rarely stops on its own and may stop until after treatment. Persistent atrial fibrillation is a condition in which the atrial fibrillation continues more than 7 days. This type of atrial fibrillation may or may not stop with treatment. Permanent atrial fibrillation is a condition in which the sinus rhythm cannot be converted with treatments. Both paroxysmal and persistent atrial fibrillation may become more frequent and eventually result in permanent atrial fibrillation. In this ECG, the atrial fibrillation stops abruptly and converts to sinus rhythm (see Fig. 74-1), therefore most likely paroxysmal.

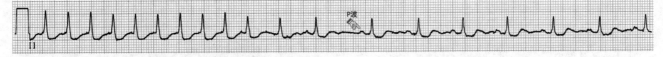

图74-1　阵发性心房颤动终止和窦性心律恢复

Fig. 74-1　Paroxysmal atrial fibrillation ends and converts to sinus rhythm

图例 75　心房颤动

Case 75　Atrial Fibrillation

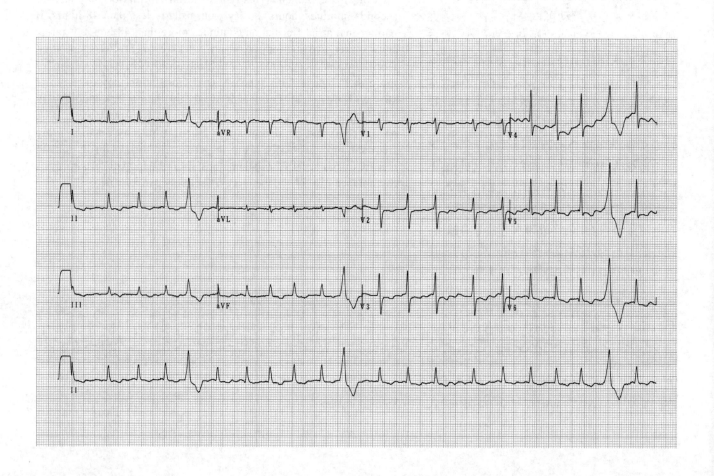

心电图特点

1. 心率：126次/min；PR间期：/；QRS波时间：98 ms；QT/QTc间期：310/448 ms；QRS波电轴：59°。

2. P波消失，代之以f波。f波快速而且不规则。心室率快速而且节律绝对不规则。可见三个宽QRS波。

心电图诊断与解析

诊断：心房颤动；室性早搏。

解析：解释心房颤动中出现宽QRS波时，应该考虑QRS波形态、前周期和联律间期等问题。宽QRS波呈右束支阻滞形态（V1导联呈rsR′型，V6导联可见宽S波），前周期长，以及联律间期短，强烈提示心室内差异传导。此心电图上，宽QRS波在V6导联呈单向R波，前周期不长，提示宽QRS波起源于心室（见图75-1）。

ECG Characteristics

1. HR: 126 bpm; PR: /; QRS D: 98 ms; QT/QTc: 310/448 ms; QRS axis: 59°.

2. The P waves are absent, replaced by small f waves. The f waves are fast and irregular. The ventricular rate is fast and the rhythm is completely irregular. There are three wide QRS complexes.

ECG Interpretation

Atrial fibrillation, ventricular premature complex.

To explain the wide QRS complex in atrial fibrillation, some considerations must be taken into account: the morphology of QRS complex, preceding interval and coupling interval. The wide QRS complex with right bundle branch block morphology (rsR′ pattern in lead V1 and broad S wave in lead V6), and with long preceding interval and short coupling interval, strongly suggests aberrant intraventricular conduction. In this ECG, the wide QRS complexes have broad R waves in lead V6 and the preceding intervals are not long, indicating that the QRS complexes originated from the ventricles (see Fig. 75-1).

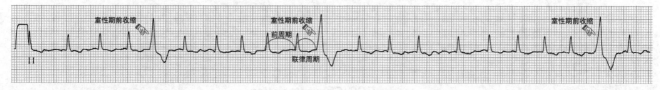

图75-1　心房颤动伴室性期前收缩

Fig. 75-1　Atrial fibrillation and ventricular premature complex

图例76 心室颤动

Case 76 Ventricular Fibrillation

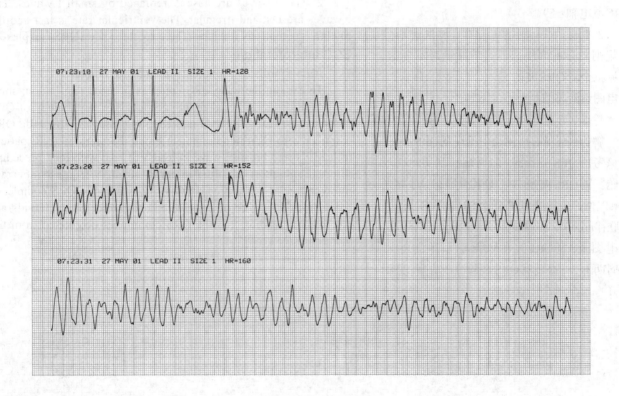

心电图特点

1. 心率：/；PR间期：/；QRS波时间：/；QT/QTc间期：/；QRS波电轴：/。

2. P–QRS–T波群消失，代之以变化不定

ECG Characteristics

1. HR: /; PR: /; QRS D: /; QT/QTc: /; QRS axis: /.

2. QRS complex, ST segment and T wave are undistinguishable replaced by unsteady and variable waves. The ventricular rate is fast and the rhythm is completely irregular.

的波。心室率快速而且节律绝对不规则。

心电图诊断与解析

诊断：心室颤动。

解析：心室扑动是非常快速（大约300次/min）而规则的心律。在心电图上类似于正弦波，无法区分QRS波、ST段和T波。心室扑动波的形态和高度是相似的。通常，非常快速的室性心动过速触发了心室扑动，然后心室扑动再触发心室颤动，除非被心脏复律治疗所终止。心室颤动是非常快速（大于300次/min）而不规则的心律。在心电图上无法识别QRS波、ST段和T波。心室颤动波的形态和高度是变化不定的。尽管如此，心室扑动和颤动之间没有明确的界线。心室扑动和颤动不能产生有效的机械运动，在短时间内将导致心脏骤停和死亡，除非立即心脏复律。此心电图上，心室颤动突然出现，并非由室性心动过速或心室扑动所触发（见图76-1）。

ECG Interpretation

Ventricular fibrillation.

Ventricular flutter is a very fast (around 300 bpm) and regular rhythm. The ECG resembles a sine-wave, without clear separation between QRS complex, ST segment and T wave. During ventricular flutter, the waves are similar in morphology and height. Usually, a very quick ventricular tachycardia triggers ventricular flutter, which then triggers ventricular fibrillation, unless it is terminated by cardioversion. Ventricular fibrillation is also a very fast (> 300 bpm) and irregular rhythm, for which the QRS complex, ST segment and T wave are undistinguishable on the ECG. During ventricular fibrillation, the waves are unsteady and variable in morphology and height. However, there are no exact borderline between ventricular flutter and fibrillation. Ventricular flutter or fibrillation does not generate effective mechanical activity and leads to cardiac arrest and death in a short period of time, unless the patient undergoes cardioversion immediately. In this ECG, ventricular fibrillation appears suddenly and is not triggered by ventricular tachycardia or flutter (see Fig. 76-1).

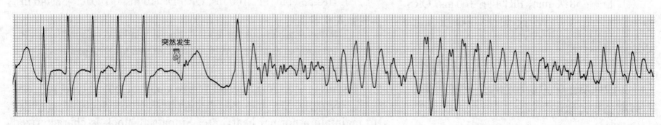

图76-1　心室颤动突然发生

Fig. 76-1　Ventricular fibrillation appears suddenly

图例77 二度Ⅰ型窦房阻滞

Case 77 Second Degree Sinoatrial Block, Type Ⅰ

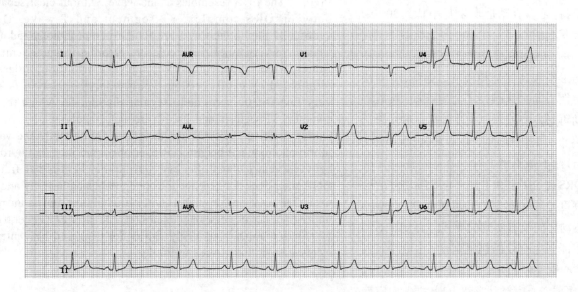

心电图特点

1. 心率: 58次/min; PR间期: 160 ms; QRS波时间: 110 ms; QT/QTc间期: 458/446 ms; QRS波电轴: 45°。

2. P波在Ⅰ和Ⅱ导联直立,在aVR导联倒置。

3. PP间期逐渐缩短,直至出现一长PP间期。

心电图诊断与解析

诊断: 窦性心动过缓; 二度Ⅰ型窦房阻滞。

解析: 正常时,窦房结产生和传导冲动来

ECG Characteristics

1. HR: 58 bpm; PR: 160 ms; QRS D: 110 ms; QT/QTc: 458/446 ms; QRS axis: 45°.

2. P waves are upright in leads Ⅰ and Ⅱ, and inverted in lead aVR.

3. PP intervals progressively shorten, until a long PP pause occurs.

ECG Interpretation

Sinus bradycardia, second degree sinoatrial block, type Ⅰ.

Normally, the sinus node generates and conducts the impulse to maintain a normal heart rate. Sinoatrial block is characterized by a transient failure of impulse conduction to the atria. Sinoatrial block may be classified into first (delay in conduction), second

维持正常的心率。窦房阻滞的特点是冲动向心房传导异常。窦房阻滞可以分成一度(传导延迟)、二度(间歇性阻滞)和三度(完全阻滞),然而心电图只能诊断二度窦房阻滞。一度窦房阻滞是冲动延迟到达心房,心电图不能发现窦房结电活动和传导延迟,因此不能诊断。三度窦房阻滞时没有冲动到达心房,在心电图上无P-QRS-T波群,或交界性或室性逸搏心律成为主导心律,因此无法区分三度窦房阻滞和窦性静止。二度窦房阻滞,周期性冲动向心房传导中断,在心电图上表现为间歇性长PP间期,可以被诊断。二度窦房阻滞可以分为文氏型(Ⅰ型)和莫氏型(Ⅱ型)。Ⅰ型窦房阻滞,窦房结到心房的传导时间逐渐延长,但延长增量逐渐减少,结果是PP间期逐渐缩短,直到传导中断,形成一长PP间期,长PP间期短于最短PP间期的两倍(见图77-1)。

(intermittently block) and third degree (complete block). However, only second degree S-A block can be diagnosed by ECG. In first degree sinoatrial block, the sinus impulse can reach the atria but with delay. The ECG is unable to detect sinus node activity and delay in conduction, therefore unable to diagnose. In third degree sinoatrial block, no sinus impulse conducts to atria, therefore no P-QRS-T complexes in ECG, or that A-V junctional or ventricular escape rhythm becomes the dominant rhythm. The ECG cannot distinguish cases between the third degree sinoatrial block and sinus arrest. The second degree sinoatrial block, transient failure of impulses conduction to the atrial, resulting in intermittent long PP pauses, may be detected by ECG. The second degree sinoatrial block may be of Wenckebach type (type Ⅰ) or Mobitz type (type Ⅱ). In type Ⅰ, there is a gradual lengthening of conduction time from the sinus node to the atria, but the lengthening increment is gradually less resulting in the progressive shortening of the PP interval, until a complete block initiates a long PP pause, the pause is less than twice the shortest PP interval (see Fig. 77-1).

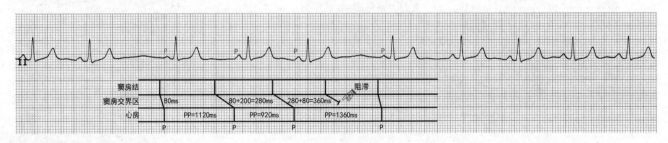

图77-1 二度Ⅰ型窦房阻滞

Fig. 77-1 Second degree sinoatrial block, type Ⅰ

图例78 二度Ⅱ型窦房阻滞

Case 78 Second Degree Sinoatrial Block, Type Ⅱ

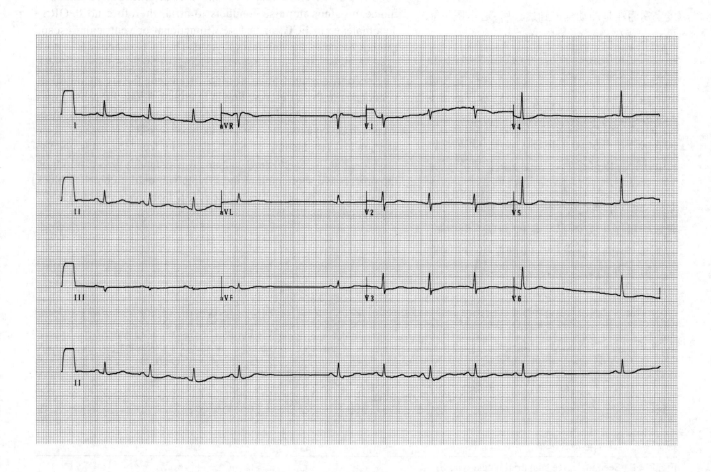

心电图特点

1. 心率：75次/min；PR间期：152 ms；QRS波时间：66 ms；QT/QTc间期：404/451 ms；QRS波电轴：45°。

2. P波在Ⅰ和Ⅱ导联直立，在aVR导联倒置。

3. PP间期恒定，可见两次长PP间期。长PP间期是短PP间期的两倍。

心电图诊断与解析

诊断：二度Ⅱ型窦房阻滞。

解析：二度Ⅱ型窦房阻滞的特点是周期性冲动向心房传导中断，形成长间期。窦房结到心房的传导时间恒定，并非逐渐延长，因此PP间期恒定。由于脱落P-QRS-T波群，窦房阻滞的长PP间期是基本节律PP间期的倍数。此心电图上，有两次长PP间期，PP间期恒定，长PP间期是短PP间期的两倍（见图78-1），诊断为二度Ⅱ型窦房阻滞。

ECG Characteristics

1. HR: 75 bpm; PR: 152 ms; QRS D: 66 ms; QT/QTc: 404/451 ms; QRS axis: 45°.

2. P waves are upright in leads Ⅰ and Ⅱ, and inverted in lead aVR.

3. The PP intervals are constant. Two long PP pauses between P waves occur. The long PP pauses are the length of two short PP intervals.

ECG Interpretation

Second degree sinoatrial block, type Ⅱ.

Second degree type Ⅱ sinoatrial block is characterized by a transient failure of impulses conduction to the atrial, resulting in intermittent long PP pauses between P waves. The conduction time from the sinus node to the atria is constant without a gradual lengthening so the PP intervals are constant. The long PP intervals including the sinoatrial block are exacted or almost exact multiples of PP intervals of the basic rhythm because of the absence of one or more beats of P-QRS-T complexes. In this ECG, there are two long PP pauses. The PP intervals are constant and the long PP pauses are almost exact multiples of the short PP intervals (see Fig. 78-1). The diagnosis is second degree sinoatrial block, type Ⅱ.

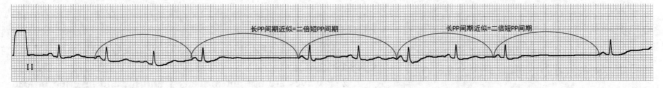

图78-1　二度Ⅱ型窦房阻滞

Fig. 78-1　Second degree sinoatrial block, type Ⅱ

图例79　二度Ⅱ型窦房阻滞，房性逸搏

Case 79　Second Degree Sinoatrial Block, Type Ⅱ, Atrial Escape Beat

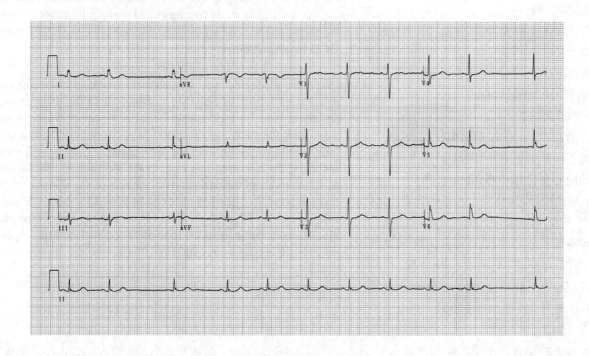

心电图特点

　　1. 心率: 71次/min; PR间期: 138 ms; QRS波时间: 88 ms; QT/QTc间期: 416/425 ms; QRS波电轴: 40°。

　　2. P波在Ⅰ和Ⅱ导联直立，在aVR导联倒置。

ECG Characteristics

　　1. HR: 71 bpm; PR: 138 ms; QRS D: 88 ms; QT/QTc: 416/425 ms; QRS axis: 40°.

　　2. P waves are upright in leads Ⅰ and Ⅱ, and inverted in lead aVR.

　　3. The PP intervals are constant. Two long PP pauses between P waves occur. The first long PP pause is the length of three short PP

3. PP间期恒定,可见两次长PP间期。第一次长PP间期是短PP间期的三倍。

4. 长PP间期中可见延迟的P'-QRS-T波群。

心电图诊断与解析

诊断:二度Ⅱ型窦房阻滞;房性逸搏。

解析:当窦性自律性降低(窦性心动过缓或窦性静止)或窦房阻滞,心率低下时,心房、房室交界区或心室的正常起搏点将发放冲动,形成逸搏或逸搏心律(被动机制)。在心电图上,逸搏是延迟的P'-QRS-T波群或QRS-T波群,前无P波。逸搏心律是指连续的逸搏(3次及以上)。此心电图上,长PP间期中,可见延迟的P'-QRS-T波群,P'波在Ⅱ导联直立,P'R间期 > 120 ms,提示逸搏起源于心房(见图79-1)。

intervals.

4. There are delayed P'-QRS-T complexes within long PP pauses.

ECG Interpretation

Second degree sinoatrial block, type Ⅱ, atrial escape beat.

With the slow heart rate as a result of depressed sinus automaticity (sinus bradycardia or sinus arrest) or sinoatrial block, an atrial, A-V junction and ventricle pacemaker may deliver one or more pacing impulses to generate escape beat and escape rhythm (passive mechanism). In ECG, the escape complex is delayed P'-QRS-T complexes or delayed QRS-T complexes not preceded by a P wave. The escape rhythm is identified as a sequence of escape beats (3 or more beats). In this ECG, there is a delayed P'-QRS-T complex within a long PP pause, the P' waves are upright in lead Ⅱ and P'R intervals are > 120 ms, suggesting that the escape beats originate from the atria (see Fig. 79-1).

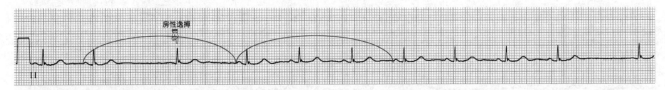

图79-1　二度Ⅱ型窦房阻滞和房性逸搏

Fig. 79-1　Second degree sinoatrial block, type Ⅱ and atrial escape beat

图例80　二度Ⅱ型窦房阻滞，交界性逸搏

Case 80　Second Degree Sinoatrial Block, Type Ⅱ, A–V Junctional Escape Beat

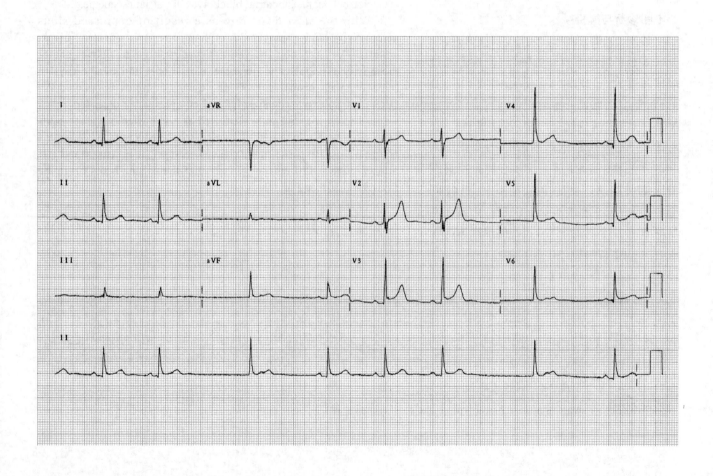

心电图特点

1. 心率: 62次/min; PR间期: 178 ms; QRS波时间: 89 ms; QT/QTc间期: 414/420 ms; QRS波电轴: 53°。

2. P波在Ⅰ和Ⅱ导联直立, 在aVR导联倒置。

3. PP间期恒定, 可见两次长PP间期。长PP间期是短PP间期的两倍。

4. 长PP间期中可见延迟的QRS-T波群, QRS波形态正常。

心电图诊断与解析

诊断: 二度Ⅱ型窦房阻滞; 交界性逸搏。

解析: 此心电图上, PP间期恒定, 长PP间期是短PP间期的两倍, 长PP间期中, 可见延迟的QRS-T波群。延迟的QRS波前无P或P′波, QRS波形态正常, 提示逸搏起源于房室交界区(见图80-1)。

ECG Characteristics

1. HR: 62 bpm; PR: 178 ms; QRS D: 89 ms; QT/QTc: 414/420 ms; QRS axis: 53°.

2. P waves are upright in leads Ⅰ and Ⅱ, and inverted in lead aVR.

3. The PP intervals are constant. Two long PP pauses between P waves occur. The long PP pauses are the length of two short PP intervals.

4. There are delayed QRS-T complexes within long PP pauses and the morphology of QRS complex is normal.

ECG Interpretation

Second degree sinoatrial block, type Ⅱ, A-V junctional escape beat.

In this ECG, the PP intervals are constant and the long PP pauses are the length of two short PP intervals. There are delayed QRS-T complexes within long PP pauses and the delayed QRS-T complexes are not preceded by a P or P′ wave and the morphology of QRS complex is normal, suggesting that the escape beats originate from the A-V junction (see Fig. 80-1).

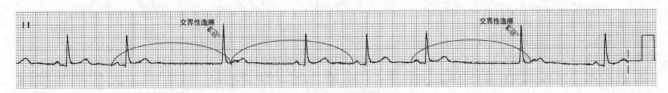

图80-1　二度Ⅱ型窦房阻滞和交界性逸搏

Fig. 80-1　Second degree sinoatrial block, type Ⅱ; A-V junctional escape beat

图例81　一度房室传导阻滞

Case 81　First Degree A-V Block

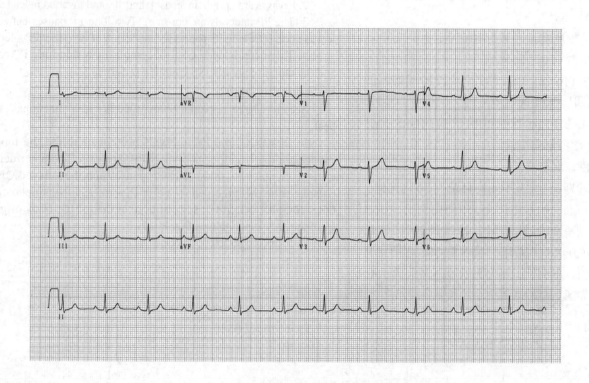

心电图特点

1. 心率: 65次/min; PR间期: 204 ms; QRS波时间: 92 ms; QT/QTc间期: 390/405 ms; QRS波电轴: 90°。

2. P波在Ⅰ和Ⅱ导联直立, 在aVR导联

ECG Characteristics

1. HR: 65 bpm; PR: 204 ms; QRS D: 92 ms; QT/QTc: 390/405 ms; QRS axis: 90°.

2. P waves are upright in leads Ⅰ and Ⅱ, and inverted in lead aVR.

3. QRS complexes are upright in leads Ⅰ, Ⅱ and in left precordial leads (V5, V6), and inverted in leads aVR and V1; QRS

倒置。

3. QRS波在 Ⅰ 、Ⅱ 和左胸导联主波向上，在aVR和V1导联主波向下，胸前导联由主波向下转为主波向上。

4. PR间期延长至 > 200 ms，每个P波后均有QRS波，PR间期恒定。

心电图诊断与解析

诊断：窦性心律；一度房室传导阻滞。

解析：房室传导阻滞是心脏传导阻滞中的常见类型。房室传导阻滞的特点是心房冲动向心室传导异常，原因是房室交界区和（或）双侧束支系统不应期延长。房室传导阻滞可以是延迟、间歇性或完全性，分别对应为一度、二度和三度。一度房室传导阻滞是心房冲动延迟到达心室，通常阻滞发生在房室结，结果是PR间期延长至 > 200 ms，但每个P波后均有QRS波，PR间期恒定(见图81-1)。

complexes change from mainly negative to mainly positive in the precordial leads.

4. The PR intervals prolong to > 200 ms, a QRS complex follows each P wave, and the PR intervals remain constant.

ECG Interpretation

Sinus rhythm, first degree A–V block.

A–V block is most common among the heart blocks. A–V block is characterized by an abnormal conduction of atrial impulses to the ventricles due to a prolonged refractory period in the A–V junctional tissue and/or bilateral bundle branch system. A–V conduction can be delayed, intermittently blocked, or completely blocked, classified correspondingly as first, second, or third degree block. In first degree block, there is a delay in the conduction of the atrial impulse to the ventricles, usually at the level of the A–V node. This results in prolongation of the PR interval to > 200 ms. A QRS complex follows each P wave, and the PR intervals remain constant (see Fig. 81–1).

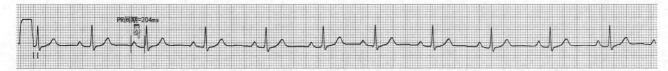

图81-1　一度房室传导阻滞

Fig. 81-1　First degree A–V block

图例82 一度房室传导阻滞

Case 82　First Degree A–V Block

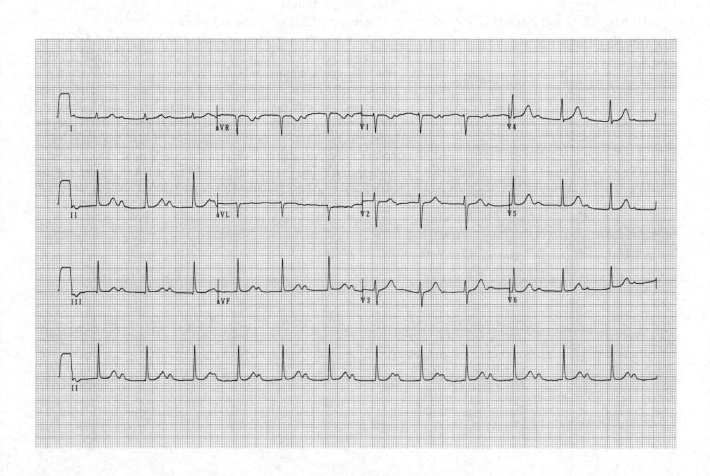

心电图特点

1. 心率：75次/min；PR间期：422 ms；QRS波时间：82 ms；QT/QTc间期：374/417 ms；QRS波电轴：85°。

2. P波在Ⅰ和Ⅱ导联直立，在aVR导联倒置。

3. QRS波在Ⅰ、Ⅱ和左胸导联主波向上，aVR和V1导联主波向下，胸前导联由主波向下转为主波向上。

4. PR间期延长至 > 200 ms，每个P波后均有QRS波，PR间期恒定。

心电图诊断与解析

诊断：窦性心律；一度房室传导阻滞。

解析：此心电图房室传导阻滞的特点是PR间期非常长，但每个P波后均有QRS波，PR间期恒定（见图82-1），心电图诊断是一度房室传导阻滞。

ECG Characteristics

1. HR: 75 bpm; PR: 422 ms; QRS D: 82 ms; QT/QTc: 374/417 ms; QRS axis: 85°.

2. P waves are upright in leads Ⅰ and Ⅱ, and inverted in lead aVR.

3. QRS complexes are upright in leads Ⅰ, Ⅱ and in left precordial leads (V5, V6), and inverted in leads aVR and V1; QRS complexes change from mainly negative to mainly positive in the precordial leads.

4. The PR intervals prolong to > 200 ms, a QRS complex follows each P wave, and the PR intervals remain constant.

ECG Interpretation

Sinus rhythm, first degree A–V block.

In this ECG, the characteristic of the A–V block is that the PR interval is very long, but a QRS complex follows each P wave, and the PR intervals remain constant (see Fig. 82-1). The ECG interpretation is first degree A–V block.

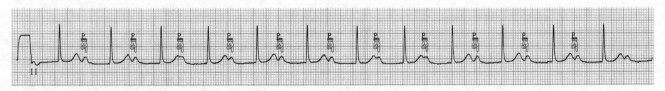

图82-1 一度房室传导阻滞

Fig. 82-1　First degree A–V block

图例83　二度Ⅰ型房室传导阻滞

Case 83　Second Degree A-V Block, Mobitz Type Ⅰ

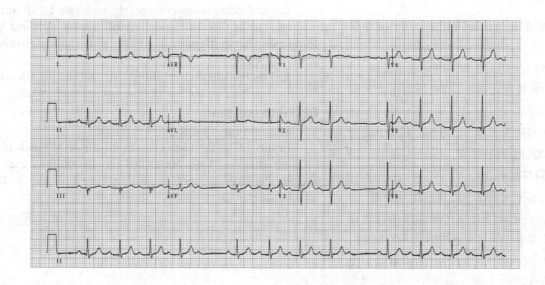

心电图特点

1. 心率：心房率88次/min，心室率75次/min；PR间期：200～300 ms；QRS波时间：88 ms；QT/QTc间期：380/420 ms；QRS波电轴：13°。

2. P波在Ⅰ和Ⅱ导联直立，在aVR导联倒置。

3. QRS波在Ⅰ、Ⅱ和左胸导联主波向上，在aVR和V1导联主波向下，胸前导联由主波向下转为主波向上。

ECG Characteristics

1. HR: 88 (atrial rate) /75 (ventricular rate) bpm; PR: 200～300 ms; QRS D: 88 ms; QT/QTc: 380/420 ms; QRS axis: 13°.

2. P waves are upright in leads Ⅰ and Ⅱ, and inverted in lead aVR.

3. QRS complexes are upright in leads Ⅰ, Ⅱ and in left precordial leads (V5, V6), and inverted in leads aVR and V1; QRS complexes change from mainly negative to mainly positive in the precordial leads.

4. The PR intervals become progressively prolonged until a P wave is not followed by a QRS complex.

5. The PR interval is the shortest following a blocked P wave

4. PR间期逐渐延长,直至P波后脱落QRS波。在整个周期中,脱落后PR间期最短,脱落前PR间期最长。

心电图诊断与解析

诊断:窦性心律;二度Ⅰ型房室传导阻滞。

解析:二度房室传导阻滞,在心房和心室之间存在间歇性传导中断。一些P波后无QRS波。二度房室传导阻滞共有三种类型。Ⅰ型(也称为文氏型或莫氏Ⅰ型)是常见的类型,通常阻滞发生在房室结,产生间歇性心房向心室传导中断。在心电图上,最初的PR间期正常或轻微延长,然后PR间期逐渐延长,直至P波后脱落QRS波。随后PR间期恢复至最初的长度,呈周期性循环。因此脱落后的PR间期最短,脱落前的PR间期最长。此心电图上,最初的PR间期是200 ms,然后PR间期逐渐延长至300 ms,直至P波后脱落QRS波(见图83-1),即二度Ⅰ型房室传导阻滞。

and the longest preceding one.

ECG Interpretation

Sinus rhythm, second degree A–V block, Mobitz type Ⅰ.

In second degree block, there is intermittent failure of conduction between the atria and ventricles. Some P waves are not followed by a QRS complex. There are three types of second degree block. Type Ⅰ (also known as Wenckebach or Mobitz type Ⅰ) is the common type and block usually occurs at the A–V node, producing intermittent failure of transmission of the atrial impulse to the ventricles. In ECG, the initial PR interval is normal or slightly prolonged, and then the PR intervals become progressively prolonged until a P wave is not followed by a QRS complex. The PR interval then returns to its initial length and the cycle repeats. Therefore the PR interval is the shortest following a blocked P wave and the longest preceding one. In this ECG, the initial PR interval is 200 ms, and then the PR intervals become progressively prolonged to 300 ms, until a P wave is not followed by a QRS complex (see Fig. 83-1). This is second degree A–V block, Mobitz type.

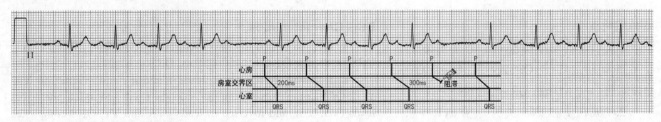

图83-1　二度Ⅰ型房室传导阻滞

Fig. 83-1　Second degree A–V block, Mobitz type Ⅰ

图例84　二度Ⅱ型房室传导阻滞

Case 84　Second Degree A–V Block, Mobitz Type Ⅱ

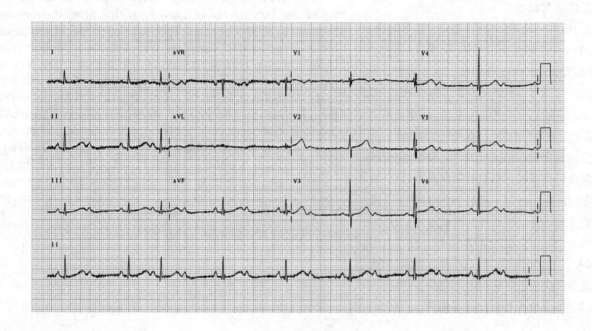

心电图特点

1. 心率：心房率88次/min，心室率46次/min；PR间期：165 ms；QRS波时间：88 ms；QT/QTc间期：460/400 ms；QRS波电轴：60°。

2. P波在Ⅰ和Ⅱ导联直立，在aVR导联倒置。QRS波在Ⅰ、Ⅱ和左胸导联主波向上，在aVR和V1导联主波向下，胸前导联由主波

ECG Characteristics

1. HR: 88 (atrial rate)/46 (ventricular rate) bpm; PR: 165 ms; QRS D: 88 ms; QT/QTc: 460/400 ms; QRS axis: 60°.

2. P waves are upright in leads Ⅰ and Ⅱ, and inverted in lead aVR. QRS complexes are upright in leads Ⅰ, Ⅱ and in left precordial leads (V5, V6), and inverted in leads aVR and V1; QRS complexes change from mainly negative to mainly positive in precordial leads. The PR intervals are constant. There is only one period in which 3 : 2

向下转为主波向上。PR间期恒定,仅一次呈
3:2传导。

心电图诊断与解析

诊断:窦性心律;二度Ⅱ型房室传导阻滞。

解析:二度Ⅱ型房室传导阻滞(也称为
莫氏Ⅱ型)是不常见类型,存在间歇性P波传
导中断。在心电图上,PR间期恒定,可以正
常或延迟,房室传导阻滞突然发生,前无PR
间期逐渐延长。阻滞常发生在双侧束支系
统,因此常伴有宽QRS波。2:1房室传导阻
滞(两个P波中一个被阻滞)难以分类,除非
出现3:2的房室传导。此心电图上,仅一周
期为3:2房室传导,能够确立二度Ⅱ型房室
传导阻滞(见图84-1)。

A-V conduction occurs.

ECG Interpretation

Sinus rhythm, second degree A-V block, Mobitz type Ⅱ.

Second degree type Ⅱ A-V block (also known as Mobitz type Ⅱ) is less common. There is intermittent failure of conduction of P waves. In ECG, the PR intervals are constant, though they may be normal or prolonged, A-V block and consequent pause occur abruptly without previous progressive prolonging of the PR intervals. The block is often at the level of the bilateral bundle branch system and is therefore associated with wide QRS complexes commonly. 2:1 A-V block (one out of two P waves is blocked) is difficult to classify, unless 3:2 A-V conduction occurs. In this ECG, there is only one period in which 3:2 A-V conduction occurs, which confirms the diagnosis of Mobitz type Ⅱ, se\cond degree A-V block (see Fig. 84-1).

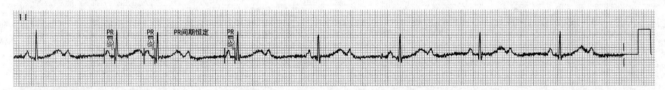

图84-1 二度Ⅱ型房室传导阻滞

Fig. 84-1 Second degree A-V block, Mobitz type Ⅱ

图例85　二度2∶1房室传导阻滞

Case 85　Second Degree 2∶1 A-V Block

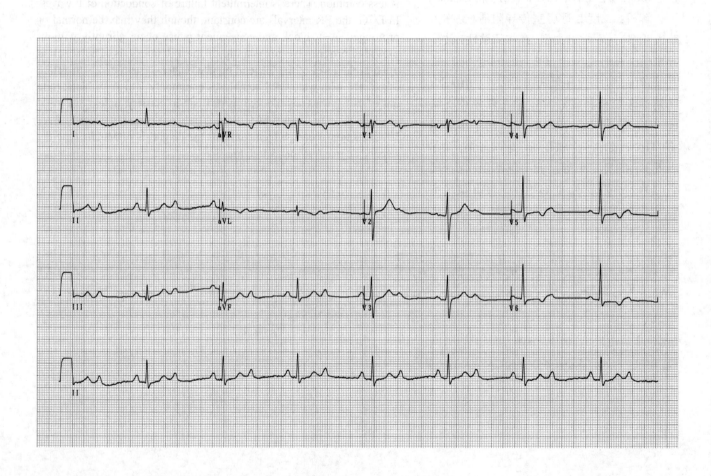

心电图特点

1. 心率：心房率92次/min，心室率46次/min；PR间期：184 ms；QRS波时间：110 ms；QT/QTc间期：460/403 ms；QRS波电轴：62°。

2. P波在Ⅰ和Ⅱ导联直立，在aVR导联倒置。

3. QRS波在Ⅰ、Ⅱ和左胸导联主波向上，在aVR和V1导联主波向下，胸前导联由主波向下转为主波向上。

4. PR间期恒定，两个P波中一个被阻滞。

心电图诊断与解析

诊断：窦性心律；二度2:1房室传导阻滞。

解析：二度房室传导阻滞，Ⅰ型和Ⅱ型之间的区别在于PR间期的变化，逐渐延长或恒定。2:1房室传导阻滞（两个P波中一个被阻滞）是特殊类型，正如此心电图所见，无法判断是何种类型（见图85-1）。

ECG Characteristics

1. HR: 92 (atrial rate)/46 (ventricular rate) bpm; PR: 184 ms; QRS D: 110 ms; QT/QTc: 460/403 ms; QRS axis: 62°.

2. P waves are upright in leads Ⅰ and Ⅱ, and inverted in lead aVR.

3. QRS complexes are upright in leads Ⅰ, Ⅱ and in left precordial leads (V5, V6), and inverted in leads aVR and V1; QRS complexes change from mainly negative to mainly positive in the precordial leads.

4. The PR intervals are constant. One out of two P waves is blocked.

ECG Interpretation

Sinus rhythm, second degree 2:1 A–V block.

In second degree A–V block, the differences between Mobitz type Ⅰ or type Ⅱ focus in whether or not the PR intervals are progressively prolonged or remain constant. 2:1 A–V block (one out of two P waves being blocked) is a peculiar case where the type is hard to be determined, as in this ECG (see Fig. 85-1).

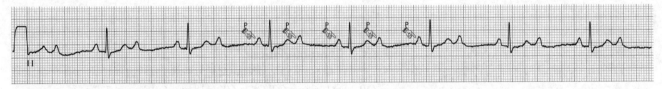

图85-1 二度2:1房室传导阻滞

Fig. 85-1 Second degree 2:1 A–V block

图例86　高度房室传导阻滞

Case 86　High Degree A–V Block

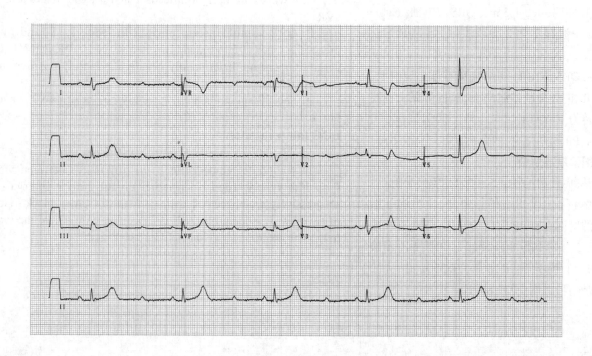

心电图特点

1. 心率：心房率88次/min，心室率46次/min；PR间期：192 ms；QRS波时间：126 ms；QT/QTc间期：600/438 ms；QRS波电轴：72°。

2. P波在Ⅰ和Ⅱ导联直立，在aVR导联倒置。

ECG Characteristics

1. HR: 88 (atrial rate)/46 (ventricular rate) bpm; PR: 192 ms; QRS D: 126 ms; QT/QTc: 600/438 ms; QRS axis: 72°.

2. P waves are upright in leads Ⅰ and Ⅱ, and inverted in lead aVR.

3. QRS complex morphology is abnormal. rsR′ pattern in lead V1, and slurred S wave in leads Ⅰ and V4 ~ V6.

4. The PR intervals are constant. Two successive P waves are

3. QRS波形态异常,V1导联呈rsR′型,Ⅰ和V4～V6导联S波粗钝。

4. PR间期恒定,连续两个P波被阻滞。

心电图诊断与解析

诊断:窦性心律;高度房室传导阻滞;完全性右束支阻滞。

解析:二度房室传导阻滞的第三种类型是高度房室传导阻滞。高度房室传导阻滞是指每三个或四个或更多P波中,仅见一个QRS波,也就是连续两个或更多P波被阻滞。这种类型的房室传导阻滞可以进展为完全性三度房室传导阻滞。此心电图上,每三个P波中,连续两个P波(其中一个P波隐入T波中)被阻滞,仅一个P波被传导,即为高度房室传导阻滞(见图86-1)。关于右束支阻滞,详见图例89。此心电图中QRS波增宽,提示阻滞位于双束支系统。

blocked.

ECG Interpretation

Sinus rhythm, high degree A–V block, complete right bundle branch block.

The third type of second degree A–V blocks is a high degree A–V block. High degree A–V block occurs when a QRS complex is seen only after every three, four, or more P waves, which means that two or more successive P waves are blocked. It may progress to a complete third degree A–V block. In this ECG, in every three P waves, two successive P waves (one of them being merged into T wave) are blocked and only one P wave is conducted, which follows the characteristics of high degree A–V block (see Fig. 86-1). The details about right bundle branch block see case 89. The QRS complexes are wide, indicating that the block is at the level of the bilateral bundle branch system.

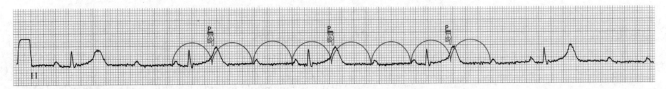

图86-1　高度房室传导阻滞

Fig. 86-1　High degree A–V block

图例87　三度房室传导阻滞，交界性逸搏心律

Case 87　Third Degree A-V Block, Junctional Escape Rhythm

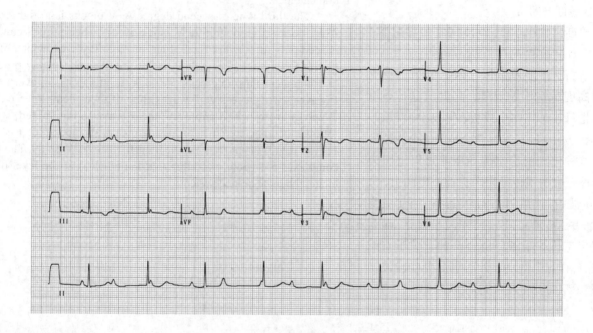

心电图特点

1. 心率：心房率78次/min，心室率50次/min；PR间期：/；QRS波时间：90 ms；QT/QTc间期：516/470 ms；QRS波电轴：79°。

2. P波在Ⅰ和Ⅱ导联直立，在aVR导联倒置。

3. QRS波在Ⅰ、Ⅱ和左胸导联主波向上，

ECG Characteristics

1. HR: 78 (atrial rate)/50 (ventricular rate) bpm; PR: /; QRS D: 90 ms; QT/QTc: 516/470 ms; QRS axis: 79°.

2. P waves are upright in leads Ⅰ and Ⅱ, and inverted in lead aVR.

3. QRS complexes are upright in leads Ⅰ, Ⅱ and in left precordial leads (V5, V6), and inverted in leads aVR and V1; QRS complex changes from mainly negative to mainly positive in the precordial leads.

aVR 和 V1 导联主波向下，胸前导联由主波向下转为主波向上。

4. P波和QRS波无关。

5. 心房率快于心室率。

心电图诊断与解析

诊断：窦性心律；三度房室传导阻滞；交界性逸搏心律。

解析：三度房室传导阻滞，心房和心室之间的传导完全中断，各自完全独立。在心电图上P波和QRS波无关。心室律依赖于阻滞远端的潜在起搏点，交界性或室性。通常心房率快于心室率。假如是交界性逸搏心律，QRS波正常，心率在40～60次/min。假如是室性逸搏心律，QRS波增宽，心率低下（15～40次/min）。此心电图中P波和QRS波无关，逸搏心律的QRS波正常，心室率50次/min，提示三度房室传导阻滞，交界性逸搏心律（见图87-1）。

4. There is a complete dissociation between the P waves and the QRS complexes.

5. The atrial rate is faster than the ventricular rate.

ECG Interpretation

Sinus rhythm, third degree A-V block, junctional escape rhythm.

In third degree block, there is a complete failure of conduction between the atria and ventricles, with complete independence of each other. There is a complete dissociation between the P waves and the QRS complexes in ECG. The ventricular rhythm is maintained by a subsidary pacemaker distal to the site of block, a junctional or a ventricular pacemaker. Usually the atrial rate is faster than the ventricular rate. A junctional escape rhythm has normal QRS complex with a rate of 40~60 bpm. A ventricular escape rhythm has wide QRS complex and is slow (15 ~ 40 bpm). In this ECG, there is a complete dissociation between the P waves and the QRS complexes and the escape rhythm has normal QRS complexes with a rate of 50 bpm, which suggest a diagnosis of third degree A-V block with junctional escape rhythm (see Fig. 87-1).

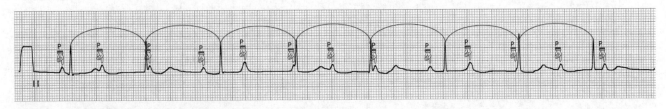

图87-1　三度房室传导阻滞伴交界性逸搏心律

Fig. 87-1　Third degree A-V block and junctional escape rhythm

图例 88 三度房室传导阻滞，室性逸搏心律

Case 88 Third Degree A–V Block, Ventricular Escape Rhythm

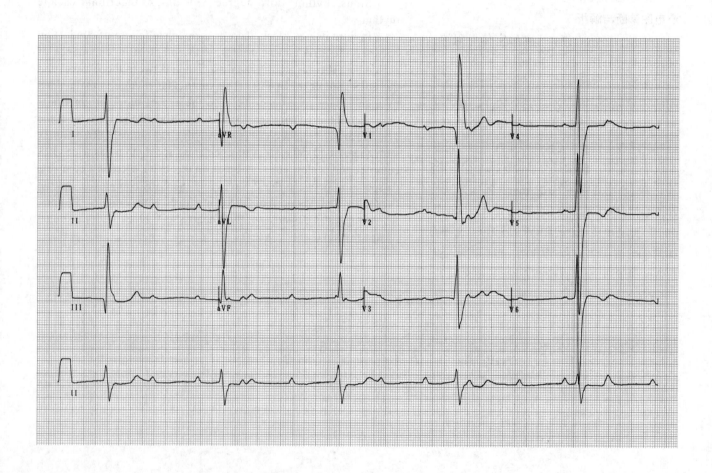

心电图特点

1. 心率：心房率77次/min，心室率30次/min；PR间期：/；QRS波时间：210 ms；QT/QTc间期：670/473 ms；QRS波电轴：155°。

2. P波在Ⅰ和Ⅱ导联直立，在aVR导联倒置。

3. QRS波形态宽大畸形。

4. P波和QRS波无关。

5. 心房率快于心室率。

心电图诊断与解析

诊断：窦性心律；三度房室传导阻滞；室性逸搏心律。

解析：此心电图中P波和QRS波无关，逸搏心律的QRS波宽大畸形，心室率30次/min，提示三度房室传导阻滞，室性逸搏心律（见图88-1）。

ECG Characteristics

1. HR: 77 (atrial rate)/30 (ventricular rate) bpm; PR: /; QRS D: 210 ms; QT/QTc: 670/473 ms; QRS axis: 155°.

2. P waves are upright in leads Ⅰ and Ⅱ, and inverted in lead aVR.

3. QRS complex morphology is wide and abnormal.

4. There is a complete dissociation between the P waves and the QRS complexes.

5. The atrial rate is faster than the ventricular rate.

ECG Interpretation

Sinus rhythm, third degree A–V block, ventricular escape rhythm.

In this ECG, there is a complete dissociation between the P waves and the QRS complexes. The escape rhythm has wide and abnormal QRS complexes with a rate of 30 bpm. The ECG interpretation is third degree A–V block with ventricular escape rhythm (see Fig. 88-1).

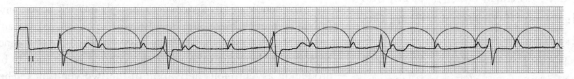

图88-1 三度房室传导阻滞伴室性逸搏心律

Fig. 88-1 Third degree A–V block and ventricular escape rhythm

图例 89   完全性右束支阻滞

Case 89   Complete Right Bundle Branch Block

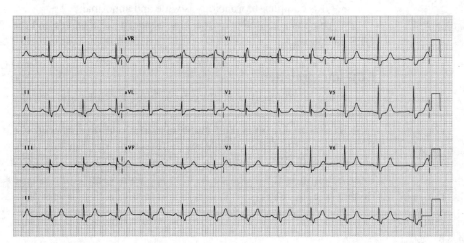

ECG Characteristics

1. HR: 73 bpm; PR: 193 ms; QRS D: 124 ms; QT/QTc: 428/472 ms; QRS axis: 130°.

2. P waves are upright in leads Ⅰ and Ⅱ, and inverted in lead aVR. QRS complex morphology is wide and abnormal. The duration of the QRS complex is > 120 ms. A secondary R wave (R′) occurs in lead V1 and wide slurred S waves occur in leads Ⅰ, V5, and V6. ST segment depression and T wave inversion occur in the lead V1.

心电图特点

1. 心率: 73次/min; PR间期: 193 ms; QRS 波时间: 124 ms; QT/QTc间期: 428/472 ms; QRS 波电轴: 130°。

2. P波在Ⅰ和Ⅱ导联直立, 在aVR导联倒置。QRS波形态宽大畸形, 时间 > 120 ms。V1导联可见R′, Ⅰ、V5和V6导联S波粗钝。V1导联ST段压低, T波倒置。

心电图诊断与解析

诊断: 窦性心律; 完全性右束支阻滞。

ECG Interpretation

Sinus rhythm, complete right bundle branch block.

The bundle of His divides into the right and left bundle branches. In bundle branch block, the impulse will be conducted via an intact bundle branch so that the ventricle with a blocked bundle branch will be activated later than the ventricle with the intact bundle branch, producing asychronous activation of the two ventricles. The QRS complex is wide and abnormal. The most common and well-recognized forms of intraventricular conduction disturbances are right and left bundle branch blocks. During right bundle branch block, depolarization of the right ventricle is delayed. The left ventricle depolarizes in a normal way and the depolarization then spreads to the right ventricle through intraventricular septum, with slow depolarization of the right

解析：希氏束分为右束支和左束支。在束支阻滞中，冲动经正常侧束支传导，阻滞侧心室激动晚于正常侧心室，双侧心室不同步激动，导致QRS波宽大畸形。最常见的得到公认的心室内传导异常是左、右束支阻滞。右束支阻滞，右心室除极延迟。左心室除极正常，然后除极经室间隔向右心室传播，右心室开始自左向右的缓慢除极（见图89-1）。右束支阻滞的QRS波可以分成两部分，初始部分是未阻滞部分，其后是粗钝缓慢的阻滞部分。与此对应的是Ⅰ、V5和V6导联出现粗钝的S波和V1导联出现R'波（呈rsR'型）。QRS波时间 > 120 ms为完全性，100 ~ 110 ms为不完全性。除极异常将伴随继发性复极异常，右胸导联出现ST段压低和T波倒置。此心电图中，V1导联呈rsR'型，Ⅰ、V5和V6导联S波粗钝（见图89-2），因此是右束支阻滞。

ventricle in a left to right direction (see Fig. 89-1). The QRS complex in right bundle branch block may be divided into two parts. The first portion is the unblocked part and the second one is the blocked part that is slurred and slow. Correspondingly, it can be seen for wide and slurred S waves in leads Ⅰ, V5 and V6 and for R' wave (rsR' pattern) in lead V1. The duration of QRS complex is > 120 ms in complete and 100 ~ 110 ms in incomplete bundle branch block. Abnormal ventricular depolarization is associated with secondary repolarization changes, ST segment depression and T wave inversion in the right precordial leads. In this ECG, rsR' pattern in lead V1 and wide slurred S wave in leads Ⅰ, V5 and V6 suggest right bundle branch block (see Fig. 89-2).

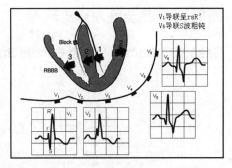

图89-1 右束支阻滞图解

Fig. 89-1 Graphic of right bundle branch block

图89-2 右束支阻滞

Fig. 89-2 Right bundle branch block

图例 90　完全性左束支阻滞

Case 90　Complete Left Bundle Branch Block

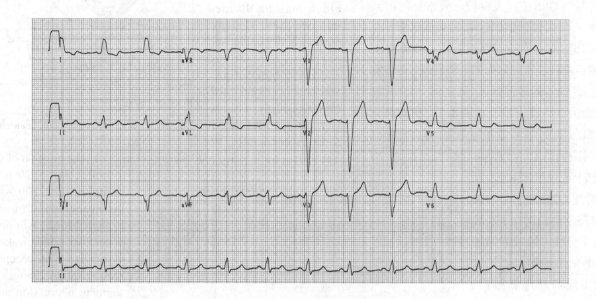

心电图特点

1. 心率：71 次/min；PR 间期：158 ms；QRS 波时间：144 ms；QT/QTc 间期：452/491 ms；QRS 波电轴：−17°。

2. P 波在 Ⅰ 和 Ⅱ 导联直立，在 aVR 导联倒置。QRS 波形态宽大畸形，时间 > 120 ms。Ⅰ、V5 和 V6 导联可见单向宽大的 R 波，V5 和 V6 导联无 Q 波。V1 ~ V3 导联宽大的 rS 波。

ECG Characteristics

1. HR: 71 bpm; PR: 158 ms; QRS D: 144 ms; QT/QTc: 452/491 ms; QRS axis: −17°.

2. P waves are upright in leads Ⅰ and Ⅱ, and inverted in lead aVR. QRS complex morphology is wide and abnormal. The duration of the QRS complex is > 120 ms. Broad monophasic R waves occur in leads Ⅰ, V5, and V6. Q waves absent in leads V5 and V6. Broad rS waves occur in leads V1 ~ V3. ST segments depression and T waves inversion occur in leads Ⅰ, aVL and V4 ~ V6. ST segments elevation and positive T waves occur in leads V1 ~ V3.

Ⅰ、aVL 和 V4 ~ V6 导联 ST 段压低，T 波倒置。V1 ~ V3 导联 ST 段抬高，T 波直立。

心电图诊断与解析

诊断：窦性心律；完全性左束支阻滞。

解析：正常时，室间隔由左向右除极，在左胸导联形成 Q 波。在左束支阻滞中，心室内室间隔除极翻转，左心室除极延迟，左胸导联 Q 波消失，代之以宽大的单向 R 波（见图 90-1）。心室除极异常，使 QRS 波时间延长至 > 120 ms。除极异常将伴随继发性复极异常，R 波为主的导联（Ⅰ、aVL 和 V4 ~ V6）出现 ST 段压低和 T 波倒置，S 波为主的导联（V1 ~ V3 导联）出现 ST 段抬高和 T 波直立。本心电图中，Ⅰ、V5 和 V6 导联可见单向宽大的 R 波，V1 ~ V3 导联可见宽大的 rS 波，V5 和 V6 导联无 Q 波，因此是左束支阻滞（见图 90-2）。

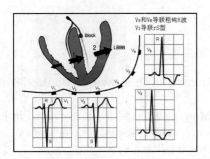

图 90-1　左束支阻滞图解

Fig. 90-1　Graphic of left bundle branch block

ECG Interpretation

Sinus rhythm, complete left bundle branch block.

Normally, septal depolarization proceeds from left to right, producing Q wave in the left precordial leads. In left bundle branch block, the direction of depolarization of the intraventricular septum is reversed and depolarization of the left ventricle is delayed. Q wave absent and replaced with a broad monophasic R waves in the left precordial leads (see Fig. 90-1). The delay in left ventricular depolarisation increases the duration of the QRS complex to > 120 ms. Abnormal ventricular depolarization leads to secondary repolarization changes. ST segments depression and T waves inversion are seen in leads with a dominant R waves (leads Ⅰ, aVL and V4~V6). ST segments elevation and positive T waves are seen in leads with a dominant S waves (leads V1~V3). In this ECG, duration of the QRS complex is > 120 ms. There are broad monophasic R waves in leads Ⅰ, V5, and V6, and broad rS waves in leads V1~V3, and an absence of Q waves in leads V5 and V6. Therefore, ECG interpretation is left bundle branch block (see Fig. 90-2).

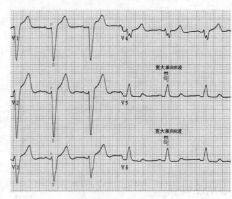

图 90-2　左束支阻滞

Fig. 90-2　Left bundle branch block

图例91　左前分支阻滞

Case 91　Left Anterior Fascicular Block

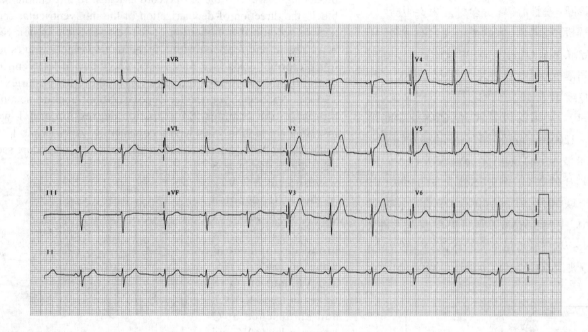

心电图特点

1. 心率：70次/min；PR间期：131 ms；QRS波时间：86 ms；QT/QTc间期：356/384 ms；QRS波电轴：−45°。

2. P波在Ⅰ和Ⅱ导联直立，在aVR导联倒置。aVL导联呈qR型，aVL导联R峰值>45 ms。Ⅱ、Ⅲ和aVF导联呈rS型。

ECG Characteristics

1. HR: 70 bpm; PR: 131 ms; QRS D: 86 ms; QT/QTc: 356/384 ms; QRS axis: −45°.

2. P waves are upright in leads Ⅰ and Ⅱ, and inverted in lead aVR. The qR pattern occurs in lead aVL, R-peak time in lead aVL is > 45 ms. The rS patterns in leads Ⅱ, Ⅲ and aVF.

ECG Interpretation

Sinus rhythm, left anterior fascicular block.

心电图诊断与解析

诊断：窦性心律；左前分支阻滞。

解析：左束支分为左前分支和左后分支。左前和左后分支阻滞，阻滞区域除极延迟，心室除极顺序发生改变。分支阻滞后，主要征象是额面QRS波变形。由于延迟激动在单个心腔内，不存在经室间隔的延迟，因此QRS波时间<120 ms。左前分支阻滞时，最初的电势来自右心室、室间隔中部和左心室后乳头肌的总和，QRS波初始电势指向右下方。随后，左心室下壁和心尖部除极，最后左心室侧壁和前壁除极。这些部位的除极形成了第二个主要电势指向左上方。在心电图上，主要表现为额面电轴左偏，aVL导联呈qR型，Ⅱ、Ⅲ和VF导联呈rS型。左前分支阻滞的诊断标准包括：电轴左偏，在−45°～−90°之间，aVL导联呈qR型，aVL导联R峰值＞45 ms，QRS波时间<120 ms（见图91-1）。

The left bundle branch splits into anterior and posterior hemifascicles. Hemiblocks occurring in the left anterior or posterior hemifascicles cause the blocked zone to depolarize later, changing the sequence of left ventricular depolarization. A major sign of hemiblocks is QRS complex modification mainly in the frontal plane. Because activation delay is only intraventricular and not transseptal, it does not produce a QRS complex of 120 ms or more. In left anterior fascicular block, the first force represents the sum of depolarization of part of the right ventricle, the medial third of the septum and the area of the left ventricular posterior papillary muscle. The QRS complex begins with a force directed to the right and downward. Later, ventricular depolarizes the lower left ventricular wall and apex, and finally, the lateral and anterior wall of the left ventricle. This produces a second powerful force directed to the left and upward. In ECG, it is manifested as frontal plane axis upward and leftward deviation, qR pattern in lead aVL, and rS pattern in leads Ⅱ, Ⅲ and aVF. Diagnostic criteria of left anterior fascicular block include that frontal plane axis between −45° ～ −90°, qR pattern in lead aVL, R-peak time in lead aVL of 45 ms or more, and QRS duration less than 120 ms (see Fig. 91-1).

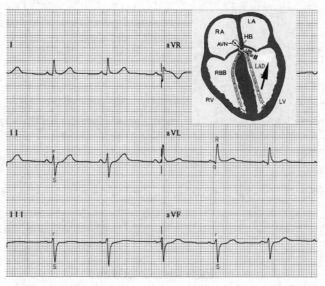

图91-1 左前分支阻滞

Fig. 91-1 Left anterior fascicular block

注：RA：右心房；RV：右心室；LA：左心房；LV：左心室；AVN：房室；HB：希氏束；LBB：左束支；RBB：右束支；LAD：电轴左偏

图例92　左后分支阻滞

Case 92　Left Posterior Fascicular Block

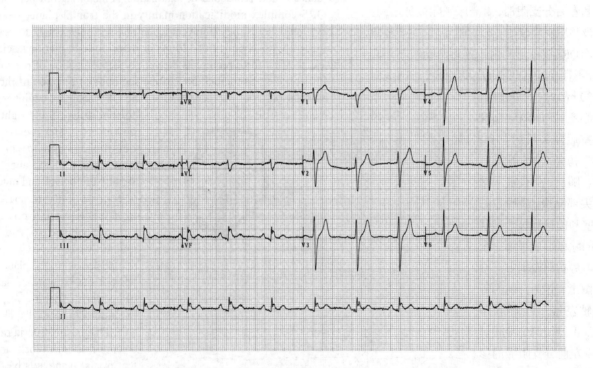

心电图特点

1. 心 率: 68次/min, PR间 期: 186 ms, QRS波时间: 120 ms, QT/QTc间期: 362/384 ms, QRS波电轴: 90°。

2. P波在Ⅰ和Ⅱ导联直立, 在aVR导联

ECG Characteristics

1. HR: 68 bpm; PR: 186 ms; QRS D: 120 ms; QT/QTc: 362/384 ms; QRS axis: 90°.

2. P waves are upright in leads Ⅰ and Ⅱ, and inverted in lead aVR. The rS patterns occur in leads Ⅰ and aVL. The qR patterns occur in leads Ⅲ and aVF.

倒置。Ⅰ和aVL导联呈rS型。Ⅲ和aVF导联呈qR型。

心电图诊断与解析

诊断：窦性心律；左后分支阻滞。

解析：左后分支阻滞时，最初的电势来自左心室前乳头肌和室间隔中部，QRS波初始电势指向左前和上方。在此左心室前壁除极，最后是阻滞区域的左心室下侧壁除极。这部位的除极形成了第二个主要电势指向右后和下方。左后分支阻滞的诊断标准包括：成人额面电轴右偏在90°～180°，Ⅰ和aVL导联呈rS型，Ⅲ和aVF导联呈qR型，QRS波时间<120 ms（见图92-1）。

ECG Interpretation

Sinus rhythm, left posterior fascicular block.

In posterior fascicular block, the first force presents the depolarization of the zone corresponding to the anterior papillary muscle of the left ventricle and of the middle third of the septum. The QRS complex begins with a force directed forward, upward, and to the left. From there, ventricular depolarizes the anterolateral wall of the left ventricle. Finally, the blocked zone that corresponds to the inferolateral wall of the left ventricle is depolarized. This produces a very powerful second force directed to the right, backward, and downward. Diagnostic criteria of left posterior fascicular block include: frontal plane axis between 90°～180° in adults, rS pattern in leads Ⅰ and aVL, qR pattern in leads Ⅲ and aVF, and QRS duration less than 120 ms (see Fig. 92-1).

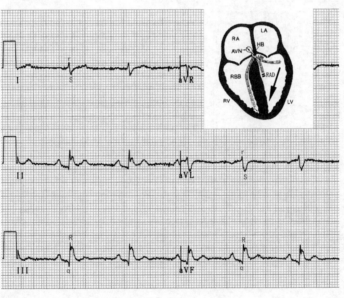

图92-1　左后分支阻滞

Fig. 92-1　Left posterior fascicular block

注：RA：右心房；RV：右心室；LA：左心房；LV：左心室；AVN：房室；HB：希氏束；LBB：左束支；RBB：右束支；RAD：电轴右偏

图例93 不定型心室内阻滞

Case 93 Nonspecific Intraventricular Conduction Disturbance

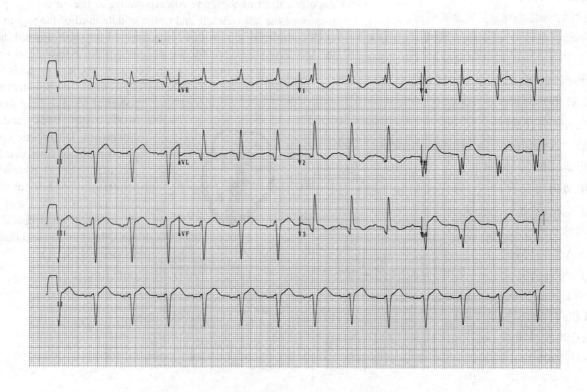

心电图特点

1. 心率: 79次/min; PR间期: 194 ms; QRS波时间: 168 ms; QT/QTc间期: 406/466 ms; QRS波电轴: −80°。

ECG Characteristics

1. HR: 79 bpm; PR: 194 ms; QRS D: 168 ms; QT/QTc: 406/466 ms; QRS axis: −80°.

2. P waves are upright in leads I and II, and inverted in lead aVR. The QRS complexes is wide and abnormal.

2. P波在Ⅰ和Ⅱ导联直立，在aVR导联倒置。QRS波宽大畸形。

心电图诊断与解析

诊断：窦性心律；不定型心室内阻滞。

解析：心室内激动普遍延迟，称为不定型心室内阻滞。在心电图上表现为QRS波增宽 > 110 ms，不符合任何类型束支阻滞的图形。同样，若胸前导联呈右束支阻滞图形，而肢体导联呈左束支阻滞图形，或反之，也称为不定型心室内阻滞。这类异常心电图主要见于慢性缺血性心脏病和心肌病。本心电图是一例心肌病的患者，QRS波增宽，不符合任何类型束支阻滞的图形，心电图诊断为不定型心室内阻滞（见图93-1）。

ECG Interpretation

Sinus rhythm, nonspecific intraventricular conduction disturbance.

Delayed diffuse intraventricular activation is termed as nonspecific or unspecified intraventricular conduction disturbance. In ECG, it manifest as QRS duration >110 ms without any ECG pattern of bundle branch block. The definition may also be applied to a pattern with right bundle branch block criteria in the precordial leads and left bundle branch block criteria in the limb leads, and vice versa. This type of abnormal ECG has been found especially in patients with chronic ischemic heart disease or cardiomyopathy. This ECG is an example of a case with cardiomyopathy. The QRS complexes are wide and abnormal without any ECG pattern of bundle branch block, so it is nonspecific intraventricular conduction disturbance (see Fig. 93-1).

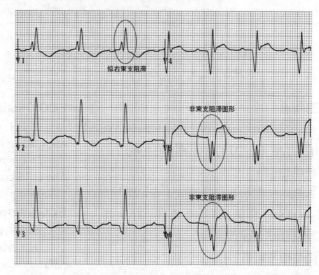

图93-1　不定型心室内阻滞

Fig. 93-1　Nonspecific intraventricular conduction disturbance

图例94　心室预激

Case 94　Ventricular Pre-excitation

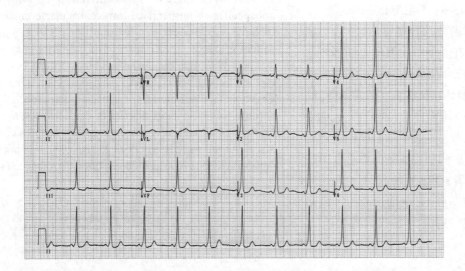

心电图特点

1. 心率：69次/min；PR间期：102 ms；QRS波时间：126 ms；QT/QTc间期：434/465 ms；QRS波电轴：73°。

2. P波在Ⅰ和Ⅱ导联直立，在aVR导联倒置。QRS波增宽，起始部粗钝，有δ波。胸前导联QRS波主波向上。

心电图诊断与解析

诊断：窦性心律；心室预激

解析：在一些特定的情况下，心房冲动

ECG Characteristics

1. HR: 69 bpm; PR: 102 ms; QRS D: 126 ms; QT/QTc: 434/465 ms; QRS axis: 73°.

2. P waves are upright in leads Ⅰ and Ⅱ, and inverted in lead aVR. The QRS complexes are wide with initial slurrings (delta wave). The QRS complexes are predominantly upright in the precordial leads.

ECG Interpretation

Sinus rhythm, ventricular preexcitation.

In certain circumstances, the atrial impulse via an accessory pathway reaches the ventricles sooner than normal A–V conduction and activation of the ventricular myocardium therefore begins earlier than normal. This earlier-than-normal activation is known as "ventricular

经旁道,在正常房室传导前到达心室,心室被提前激动。这一提前的激动称之为"心室预激"。心室预激被分为三类:Wolff-Parkinson-White(WPW)、不典型和短PR心室预激。WPW是最常见的类型,提前激动经房室之间的旁道(Kent束),绕开了正常的房室结传导,在心电图上可见PR间期缩短和QRS波增宽异常,QRS波初始部位粗钝有δ波(见图94-1)。短PR间期是由于冲动经旁道传导快于经房室结传导。由于冲动进入心室肌,心室最初的激动缓慢,使得R波初始部变形,形成特征性的δ波。根据胸导联的形态,传统的WPW被分为A和B两型。A型,δ波和QRS波在胸导联上向上(见图94-2)。通常这类WPW为左侧旁道。

preexcitation". Three types of preexcitation have been defined: Wolff-Parkinson-White preexcitation (WPW), atypical preexcitation, and short PR preexcitation. WPW is the most common type in which the early excitation is caused by accessory pathways (Kent bundles) that connect the atrium and ventricle, bypassing the A–V nodal conduction. The result is that the PR interval is short and the QRS complex is wider than normal with initial slurrings (delta wave) in ECG (see Fig. 94-1). The short PR interval occurs because the impulse reaches the ventricle through the pathway sooner than through the A–V node. Because the impulse enters myocardium, ventricular activation is slowly at first, distorting the early part of the R wave and producing the characteristic delta wave. Traditionally WPW has been classified into two types according to the morphology of QRS complex in the precordial leads. In type A, the delta waves and the QRS complexes are predominantly upright in the precordial leads (see Fig. 94-2). Generally, this type is left-sided accessory pathways.

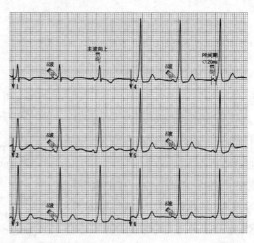

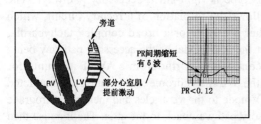

图94-1 心室预激图解

Fig. 94-1 Graphic of ventricular preexcitation

图94-2 心室预激

Fig. 94-2 Ventricular preexcitation

图例95 心室预激

Case 95　Ventricular Pre-excitation

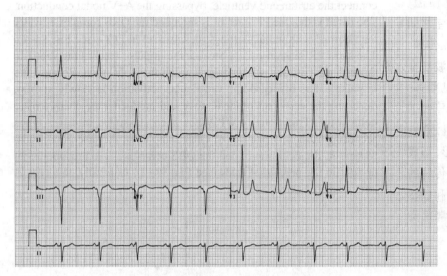

心电图特点

1. 心率: 64次/min; PR间期: 104 ms; QRS波时间: 138 ms; QT/QTc间期: 434/447 ms; QRS波电轴: −51°。

2. P波在 I 和 II 导联直立, 在aVR导联倒置。QRS波增宽, 起始部粗钝, 有 δ 波。V1导联QRS波主波向下, 其他胸前导联QRS波主波向上。

ECG Characteristics

1. HR: 64 bpm; PR: 104 ms; QRS D: 138 ms; QT/QTc: 434/447 ms; QRS axis: −51°.

2. P waves are upright in leads I and II, and inverted in lead aVR. The QRS complexes are wider with initial δ waves. The QRS complexes are predominantly negative in lead V1, and positive in the other precordial leads.

ECG Interpretation

Sinus rhythm, ventricular preexcitation.

In type B of WPW, the δ wave and QRS complex are predominantly negative in lead V1 and positive in the other precordial leads (see Fig. 95−1). Generally, this type is right-sided accessory pathways. The accessory pathway allows the formation of a reentry circuit, which may give rise to either a narrow or a broad complex tachycardia, depending on whether the A−V nodal or the accessory pathway being used for antegrade conduction. Orthodromic AVRT accounts for most tachycardia in the WPW syndrome. An impulse is conducted down through the A−V node to the ventricles and then in a retrograde fashion via the accessory pathway back to the atria. The impulse then circles repeatedly between the atria and ventricles, producing a narrow complex tachycardia. During this kind of tachycardia, the δ wave

心电图诊断与解析

诊断：窦性心律；心室预激。

解析：B型WPW，δ波和QRS波在V1导联上向下，在其他胸前导联上向上（见图95-1）。通常这类WPW为右侧旁道。旁道形成折返环，可以形成窄QRS波或宽QRS波心动过速，取决于前传是经房室结还是经旁道。顺向型AVRT是WPW综合征中最常见的心动过速。冲动经房室结前传至心室，然后经旁道逆传至心房。冲动在心房和心室之间循环折返，形成窄QRS波心动过速。心动过速中δ波不可见，QRS波形态正常。逆向型AVRT不常见，冲动经旁道前传至心室，然后经房室结逆传至心房。心动过速中可见δ波，QRS波形态异常（见图95-2）。

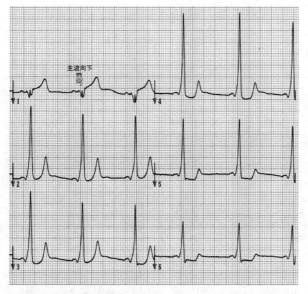

主波向下

图95-1　心室预激

Fig. 95-1　Ventricular preexcitation

cannot be observed and the QRS complex is normal. Antidromic AVRT is relatively uncommon. The accessory pathway allows antegrade conduction, and thus the impulse is conducted from the atria to the ventricles via the accessory pathways, and then in a retrograde fashion via the A–V nodal back to the atria. During this kind of tachycardia, the δ wave can be observed and the QRS complex is abnormal (see Fig. 95-2).

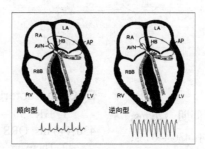

顺向型　逆向型

图95-2　心室预激与折返性心动过速

Fig. 95-2　Ventricular preexcitation and reentrant tachycardia

注: RA: 右心房; RV: 右心室; LA: 左心房; LV: 左心室; AVN: 房室; HB: 希氏束; LBB: 左束支; RBB: 右束支; AP: 旁道

图例96 房性逸搏心律

Case 96 Atrial Escape Rhythm

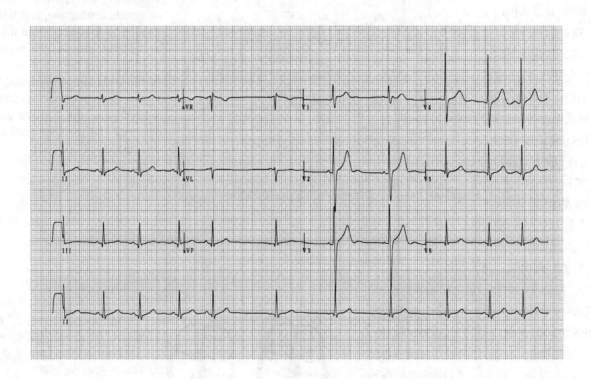

心电图特点

1. 心率: 50 ~ 75次/min; PR间期: 126 ms; QRS波时间: 94 ms; QT/QTc间期: 430/440 ms; QRS波电轴: 89°。

2. 长PP间期中可见连续的P'–QRS–T

ECG Characteristics

1. HR: 50 ~ 75 bpm; PR: 126 ms; QRS D: 94 ms; QT/QTc: 430/440 ms; QRS axis: 89°.

2. There are consecutive P'–QRS–T complexes in long PP interval. P' waves are biphasic in lead II, and inverted in lead aVR.

3. QRS complexes are upright in leads I and II, and in left

波群。P′波在Ⅱ导联双向,在aVR导联倒置。

3. QRS波在Ⅰ、Ⅱ和左胸导联主波向上,在aVR和V1导联主波向下,胸前导联由主波向下转为主波向上。

心电图诊断与解析

诊断:窦性静止;房性逸搏心律。

解析:当窦性自律性降低或窦房阻滞,造成心率缓慢时,心房、交界区和心室潜在起搏点发放一个或更多冲动,起搏心脏(逸搏和逸搏心律)。在心电图上,房性逸搏的QRS波前有P′波,P′R间期 > 120 ms。此心电图上,长PP间期不是短PP间期的倍数,在长PP间期中出现连续的P′波,P′波Ⅱ导联双向,在aVR导联倒置,P′R间期 > 120 ms.(见图96-1)。在鉴别诊断上着重考虑窦性静止和房性逸搏心律。

precordial leads (V5, V6), and inverted in leads aVR and V1; QRS complex changes from mainly negative to mainly positive in precordial leads.

ECG Interpretation

Sinus arrest, atrial escape rhythm.

When the heart rate is slow as a result of depressed sinus automaticity or sinoatrial block, an atrial, A-V junction and ventricular potential pacemaker may deliver one or more electrical stimuli (escape beat or escape rhythm) to pace the heart beat. In ECG with the atrial escape beat, there is a delayed P′ wave before QRS complex, and the P′R interval is > 120 ms. In this ECG, the long PP interval is not a multiple of the short PP interval and is terminated by consecutive P′ waves. The P′ waves are biphasic in lead Ⅱ, inverted in lead aVR and the P′R intervals are > 120 ms (see Fig. 96-1). Sinus arrest and atrial escape rhythm should be the major consideration in differential diagnosis.

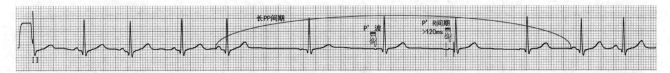

图96-1　窦性静止和房性逸搏心律

Fig. 96-1　Sinus arrest and atrial escape rhythm

图例 97　交界性逸搏心律

Case 97　Junctional Escape Rhythm

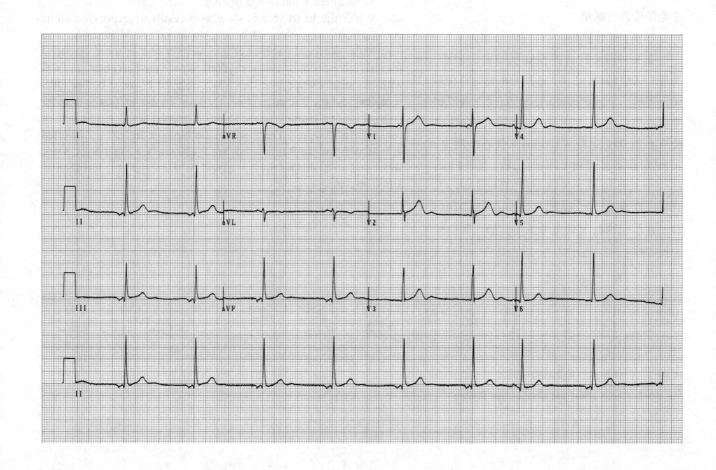

心电图特点

1. 心 率: 50次/min; PR间 期: 110 ms; QRS波时间: 82 ms; QT/QTc间期: 432/405 ms; QRS波电轴: 68°。

2. P′波在Ⅱ导联双向,在aVR导联倒置。

3. 可见一个提前的P波,P波在Ⅱ导联上直立,PR间期 > 120 ms。

4. QRS波在Ⅰ、Ⅱ和左胸导联主波向上,在aVR和V1导联主波向下,胸前导联由主波向下转为主波向上。

心电图诊断与解析

诊断: 交界性逸搏心律;窦性夺获。

解析: 逸搏心律中可以插入窦性心动,称为窦性夺获,有时夺获可形成逸搏-夺获二联律。此心电图上,逸搏心律有P′波,P′R间期<120 ms,为交界性逸搏心律。一个提前的P波插入交界性逸搏心律,为窦性夺获(见图97-1)。

ECG Characteristics

1. HR: 50 bpm; PR: 110 ms; QRS D: 82 ms; QT/QTc: 432/405 ms; QRS axis: 68°.

2. P′ waves are inverted in lead Ⅱ, and upright in lead aVR.

3. There is a premature P wave. The P wave is upright in lead Ⅱ and PR interval > 120 ms.

4. QRS complexes are upright in leads Ⅰ, Ⅱ and in left precordial leads (V5 and V6), and inverted in leads aVR and V1; QRS complex changes from mainly negative to mainly positive in precordial leads.

ECG Interpretation

Junctional escape rhythm, sinus capture beat.

The escape rhythm may be interrupted by sinus beat and it is called sinus capture. Sometimes the capture beats manifest as escape-capture bigeminy. In this ECG, there is a preceding P′ wave and the P′R interval < 120 ms in the escape rhythm, which is a junctional escape rhythm. A premature P wave interrupts the junctional escape rhythm, suggesting that this beat is sinus capture (see Fig. 97-1).

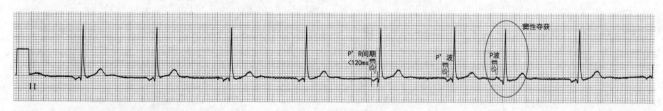

图97-1 交界性逸搏心律和窦性夺获

Fig. 97-1 Junctional escape rhythm and sinus capture beat

图例98　室性逸搏心律

Case 98　Ventricular Escape Rhythm

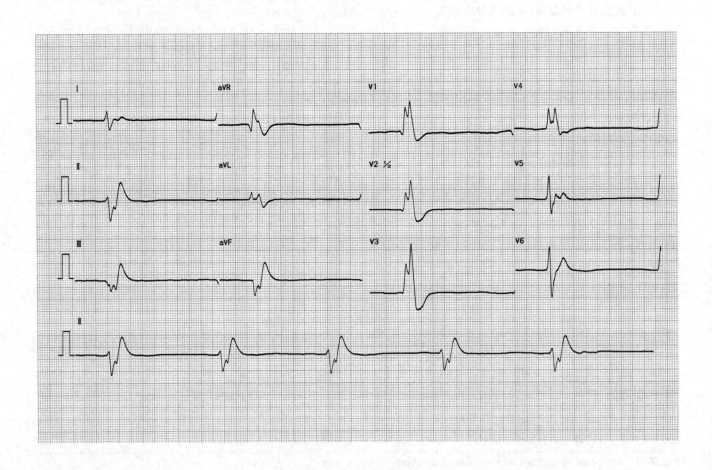

心电图特点

1. 心率：31次/min；PR间期：/；QRS波时间：200 ms；QT/QTc间期：440/316 ms；QRS波电轴：139°。

2. 缓慢的宽QRS波心律，无P或P′波。

心电图诊断与解析

诊断：室性逸搏心律

解析：此心电图上，心律由连续的宽QRS波组成，宽QRS波前无P或P′波，频率缓慢（见图98-1），诊断为室性逸搏心律。随后可能是全心停顿和死亡。

ECG Characteristics

1. HR: 31 bpm; PR: /; QRS D: 200 ms; QT/QTc: 440/316 ms; QRS axis: 139°.

2. Wide QRS complexes in slow rate without preceding P or P′ waves occur in rhythm.

ECG Interpretation

Ventricular escape rhythm.

In this ECG, the rhythm consists of consecutive wide QRS complexes. The wide QRS complexes are not preceded by P or P′ waves and the rate is slow (see Fig. 98-1). Ventricular escape rhythm should be considered as diagnosis. Cardiac standstill and death may be followed that rhythm.

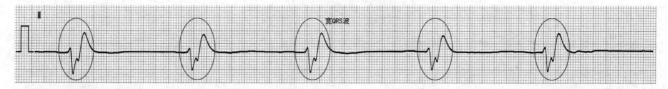

图98-1 室性逸搏心律

Fig. 98-1 Ventricular escape rhythm

图例99　提示高钾血症

Case 99　Suggestion of Hyperkalemia

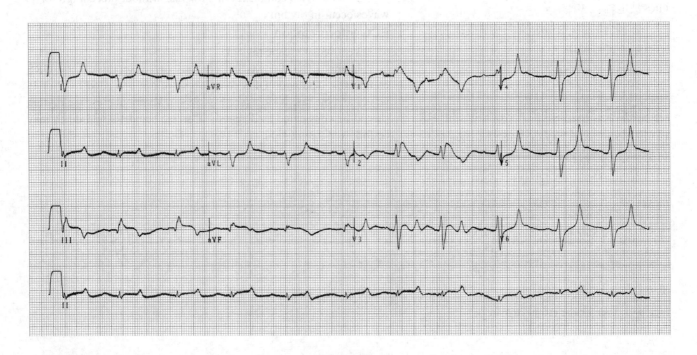

心电图特点

1. 心率：66次/min；PR间期：220 ms；QRS波时间：150 ms；QT/QTc间期：480/503 ms；QRS波电轴：148°。

2. 肢体导联上P波增宽低平。PP间期差值＞120 ms。Ⅰ、Ⅱ、aVL和V3～V6导联上

ECG Characteristics

1. HR: 66 bpm; PR: 220 ms; QRS D: 150 ms; QT/QTc: 480/503 ms; QRS axis: 148°.

2. P waves are wide and flat in limb leads. Differences between PP intervals are ＞ 120 ms in the same lead. T waves are tall, symmetrically narrow and peaked in leads Ⅰ, Ⅱ, aVL and V3 ~ V6. The PR intervals prolong and the QRS complexes are wide.

T波对称性高尖。PR间期延长，QRS波增宽。

心电图诊断与解析

诊断：提示高钾血症；窦性心律不齐；一度房室传导阻滞。

解析：高钾血症对心电图有显著的影响。与高钾血症有关的最常见的改变是T波对称性高尖、P波低平或消失和显著的QRS波增宽。最早的改变是T波增高，常见于Ⅱ、Ⅲ和V2~V4导联上。随着血钾浓度的增高，PR间期和P波发生改变，PR间期延长，P波增宽低平，或消失。随着血钾浓度的进一步增高，QRS波增宽。此心电图上，可见T波对称性高尖、PR间期延长、P波增宽低平和QRS波增宽（见图99-1），所有这些征象，提示高钾血症。此心电图是一例血钾浓度为8.3 mmol/l的患者。

ECG Interpretation

Suggestion of hyperkalaemia, sinus arrhythmia, first degree A-V block.

Hyperkalaemia may have significant effects on the ECG. The most common changes associated with hyperkalaemia are tall, symmetrically narrow and peaked T wave, reduced amplitude and eventually loss of the P wave, and marked widening of the QRS complex. The earliest changes are tall T waves, best seen in leads Ⅱ, Ⅲ, and V2~V4. As the potassium concentration rises, changes are seen in the PR interval and the P wave: the PR interval prolongs and the P wave widens and flattens or may disappear. The QRS complex will begin to widen as the concentration further rises. In this ECG, there are tall, symmetrically narrow and peaked T waves, prolonged the PR intervals, wide and flat P waves and wide QRS complexes, all these evidences suggest hyperkalaemia (see Fig. 99-1). This ECG is an example of a case with a potassium concentration of 8.3 mmol/l.

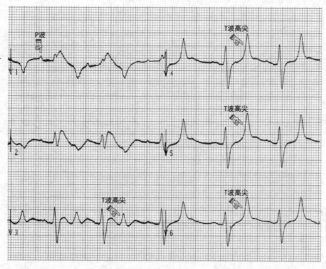

图99-1　高钾血症

Fig. 99-1　Hyperkalaemia

图例100　提示低钾血症

Case 100　Suggestion of Hypokalemia

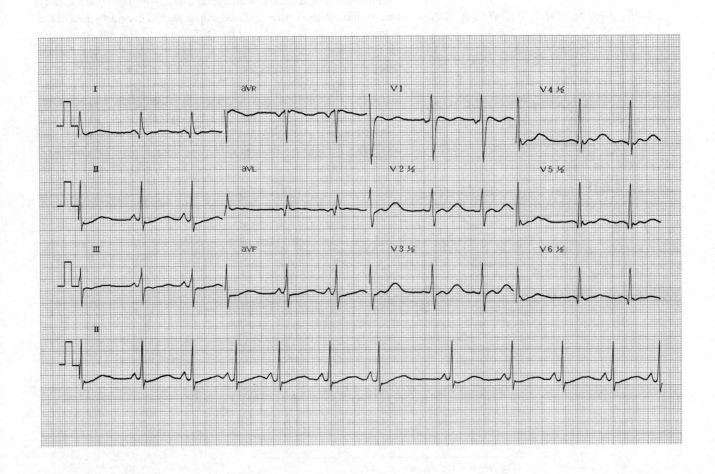

心电图特点

1. 心率：66次/min；PR间期：140 ms；QRS波时间：120 ms；QT/QTc间期：495/521 ms；QRS波电轴：57°。

2. P波在Ⅰ和Ⅱ导联直立，在aVR导联倒置。PP间期差值 > 120 ms。V2 ~ V5导联上巨大U波，T波低平。

心电图诊断与解析

诊断：提示低钾血症；窦性心律不齐。

解析：低钾血症可以造成一系列心电图改变。最常见的改变是T波振幅降低、ST段压低、出现U波和QT（QU）间期延长。巨大的U波，伴随低平的T波，是低钾血症经典的心电图改变。大部分患者看似QT间期延长，实为QU间期延长。此心电图上，V2 ~ V5导联上巨大U波、T波低平、QU间期延长（见图100-1），这些征象提示低钾血症。轻、中度低钾血症，心电图改变不常见，此心电图是一例血钾浓度为1.22 mmol/l的患者。

ECG Characteristics

1. HR: 66 bpm; PR: 140 ms; QRS D: 120 ms; QT/QTc: 495/521 ms; QRS axis: 57°.

2. P waves are upright in leads Ⅰ and Ⅱ, and inverted in lead aVR. The differences between PP intervals are > 120 ms at the same lead. A prominent U waves in association with a low T waves occur in leads V2 ~ V5.

ECG Interpretation

Suggestion of hypokalaemia, sinus arrhythmia.

Hypokalaemia may produce several ECG changes. The most common changes are decreased T wave amplitude, ST segment depression, presence of a U wave and prolonged QT (or QU) interval. A prominent U wave in association with a low T wave is considered to be the classic ECG findings of hypokalaemia. The most cases of a presumed prolongation of the QT interval are really QU intervals. In this ECG, prominent U waves are accompanied by low T waves in leads V2 ~ V5 and the QU intervals are prolonged. These evidences suggest hypokalaemia (see Fig. 100–1). The changes of ECG are not common with mild to moderate hypokalaemia. This ECG is an example of a case with a potassium concentration of 1.22 mmol/l.

图 100-1 低钾血症

Fig. 100–1 Hypokalaemia

参考文献

References

1. Hancock EW, Deal BJ, Mirvis DM, et al. AHA/ACCF/HRS Recommendations for the Standardization and Interpretation of the Electrocardiogram: Part V: Electrocardiogram Changes Associated With Cardiac, Chamber Hypertrophy: A Scientific Statement From the American Heart Association Electrocardiography and Arrhythmias Committee, Council on Clinical Cardiology; the American College of Cardiology Foundation; and the Heart Rhythm Society: Endorsed by the International Society for Computerized Electrocardiology[J]. Circulation. 2009;119: e251−e261.

2. Rautaharju PM, Surawicz B, Gettes LS, et al. AHA/ACCF/HRS Recommendations for the Standardization and Interpretation of the Electrocardiogram: Part IV: The ST Segment, T and U Waves, and the QT Interval: A Scientific Statement From the American Heart Association Electrocardiography and Arrhythmias Committee, Council on Clinical Cardiology; the American College of Cardiology Foundation; and the Heart Rhythm Society: Endorsed by the International Society for Computerized Electrocardiology[J]. Circulation. 2009;119: e241−e250.

3. Wagner GS, Macfarlane P, Wellens H, et al. AHA/ACCF/HRS Recommendations for the Standardization and Interpretation of the Electrocardiogram: Part VI: Acute Ischemia/Infarction: A Scientific Statement From the American Heart Association Electrocardiography and Arrhythmias Committee, Council on Clinical Cardiology; the American College of Cardiology Foundation; and the Heart Rhythm Society: Endorsed by the International Society for Computerized Electrocardiology[J]. Circulation. 2009;119: e262−e270.

4. Thygesen K, Alpert JS, White HD et al. Universal Definition of Myocardial Infarction[J]. Circulation. 2007;116: 2634−2653.

5. Thygesen K, Alpert JS, Jaffe AS, et al. Third Universal Definition of Myocardial Infarction[J]. Circulation. 2012;126: 2020−2035.

索　引

Index